DEMEDICALIZING WOMEN'S HEALTH

DEMEDICALIZING WOMEN'S HEALTH

(In Two Volumes)

(Volume - 2)

Editor
Dr. Amarjeet Singh

Co-Editors
Dr. (Mrs.) Indarjit Walia
Dr. Lakhbir Dhaliwal

GYAN

NEW DELHI-110002

Demedicalizing Women's Health

Rs. 1800

ISBN: 978-81-212-1019-5 (Set)
ISBN : 978-81-212-1035-5 (Vol. 2)

Published in 2010 in India by
Gyan Publishing House
Gyan Kunj 23, Main Ansari Road, Darya Ganj,
New Delhi-110002
Phones : 23282060, 23261060
Fax : 011-23285914
E-mail: books@gyanbooks.com
Website: www.gyanbooks.com

Lasser Type Setting by: Rudra Computer Graphics, Delhi
Printed at : Gian Ridhi Offset Printers, Delhi-35

Contents

21

Infertility Management - Experiences of A Private Infertility Specialist

Nirmal Bhasin

The process of reproduction is immensely complex. For conception to take place and pregnancy to be achieved, hundreds of individual hormonal, chemical and physical phenomena must occur in a precise manner.

If an infertile couple has a proper understanding of their reproductive systems, it will immensely help the doctor in obtaining their full cooperation and compliance in the treatment of infertility.

The female reproductive system comprises of the uterus (1), a pair of ovaries (2) attached to either side of the uterus. One or two eggs (3) are matured every month in each ovary to accept the sperm (4). The uterus is linked internally with fallopian tubes (5) on either side. The function of the tubes is to pick the mature egg from the ovary, where the egg waits for the sperms to reach and one of the sperms penetrates the egg and fertilization takes place in the fallopian tube. The tube with its peristaltic movement transfers the fertilized egg (embryo) (6) into the cavity of the uterus (7). When the uterus accepts the embryo; implantation takes place, which results in pregnancy. (See diagram)

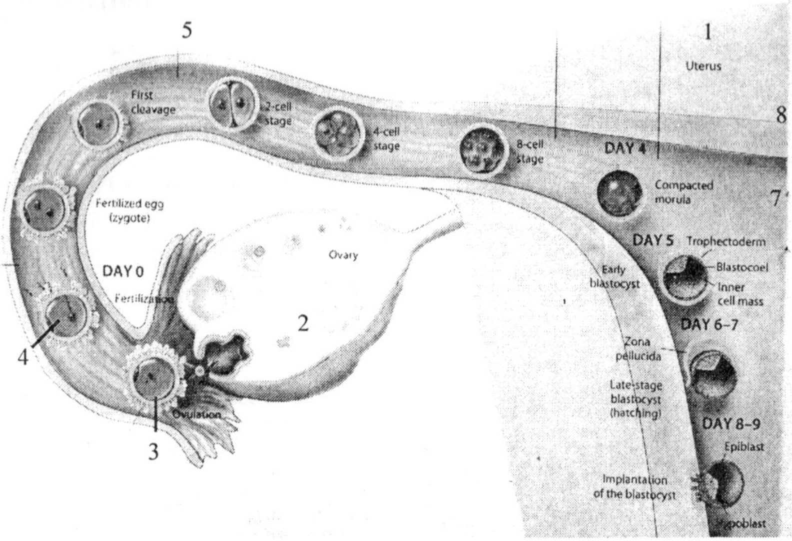

Infertility is defined as the inability to achieve pregnancy within a year by regular coital exposure. It is estimated that about 90% of couples will achieve pregnancy in the first year and 95% in two years with regular cohabitation.

Approximately, 8-10% of couples experience some kind of infertility problem worldwide. Today the graph of infertility is on the rise due to additional factors such as stress, lifestyle changes, psychosexual disorders and various forms of addictions. The abundance of treatment facilities and easy access to fertility specialists has increased the awareness amongst patients to seek medical help. Ironically, the treatment, its cost and low success rate itself aggravates the stress of infertile couples.

Few things which a couple can follow for enhancement of conception rates are listed below:

1. **TIME OF INTERCOURSE**- Coital frequency influences conception rates in the general population. Psychological stress affects libido and coital frequency and hence fertility. Sexual intercourse every 2 to 3 days optimizes the chance of pregnancy.
2. **ALCOHOL-** Women trying to conceive should avoid alcohol as it increases the risk of harming the developing fetus. Excessive alcohol intake is detrimental to semen quality in men.

3. **SMOKING**- There is an association between smoking and reduced semen quality and quitting improves sperm count & motility. For women not only active smoking but even passive smoking is likely to affect their fertility.
4. **EXCESSIVE BODY WEIGHT** (Obesity) - BMI (body mass index) is a measure of body fat calculated from an individual's weight and height (kg/meter square). With BMI over 29 kg/ meter sq, the recommendations are to lose weight and include exercise and diet program in the lifestyle. Men who are obese may have erectile dysfunction, risk of heart disease or diabetes leading to low sperm count.
5. **TIGHT UNDERWEAR FOR MEN**- Nature has located the testes in the scrotum outside the body of the male because the development of sperms requires a temperature which is about 2 degree lower than the internal body temperature (30 to 34 degree Celsius). High temperature, sedentary work position and tight briefs bring the testes closer to the body hence increasing the temperature to 37 degree Celsius (body temperature). This leads to reduced sperm count and motility.
6. **OCCUPATION**- Some occupations involve exposure to hazards and evidence of harmful effects on human reproductive system has been recognized for specific agents as heat, x-rays, metals, pesticides, paints.
7. **DRUG ABUSE-Prescribed drug abuse**- Indiscriminate use of anti-inflammatory drugs, antidepressants, tranquilizers or asthma medication affect the ovulation (egg formation) in females. Immunosuppressive drugs used in rheumatic disease may affect conception. Chemotherapy can induce ovarian failure in women and azoospermia (absence of sperms) in man.

   Recreational drug abuse- Marijuana, cocaine, opium adversely affects ovulatory and tubal functions in women and maturation of sperms in men.
8. **MULTIPLE SEX PARTNERS**- The practice of multiple sex partners promotes the spread of sexually transmitted diseases. This leads to infections of the reproductive organs and total damage to the tubules in females and sperm quality in males.

Factors influencing infertility:

In 40% cases of infertility female factors are involved.

(1) Tubal Block- The fallopian tubes may be blocked due to infections, e.g tuberculosis, sexually transmitted diseases leading to pelvic inflammation, repeated abortions.

(2) Ovulatory dysfunctions- The egg may not be released due to hormonal imbalance e.g. polycystic ovarian syndrome.

(3) Psychosexual disorders – The couple may not be able to have sexual intercourse properly due to vaginismus or fear of penetration, decreased libido.

(4) Endometriosis.

(5) Alcohol and drug abuse.

(6) Unexplained infertility (mainly related to stress).

In 30% cases male factors are involved.

(1) Oligoasthenospermia - Decreased sperm count and decreased motility.

(2) Spinal injuries.

(3) Congenital bilateral absence of Vas Deferens (CBAVD).

(4) Obstructive azoospermia -Absence of sperms due to blockage, which can be corrected with surgery.

(5) Chronic alcoholism, smoking and drug abuse-reduces the sperm quantity and quality.

(6) Psychosexual disorders (erectile dysfunctions, decreased libido).

In rest 30% cases combined factors are involved - both in the male and the female partner.

Tubal factor: For sometime, during the "sexual revolution" of the 1960's and 70's doctors did see a higher incidence of infertility caused by tubal blockages left by untreated venereal diseases such as gonorrhea, chlamydia, and syphilis. Today, approximately 30% of tubal blockages are caused by mycobacterium tuberculosis, which was undiagnosed and untreated in the yesteryears.

Personal hygiene of the intimate parts reduces infections caused to the pelvic organs. Education of the girl child should begin at a very tender age by cultivating the habit of cleaning private parts with soap and water at least twice a day apart from washing with water after every bowel movement. Today, the prevention of pelvic organ infections is simple with the easy availability of special feminine wash soaps containing lactic acid (Lactimark, Lactacyd).

They help in retaining the vaginal pH, which helps in the growth of the lactic acid bacillus, the healthy bacteria in the vagina responsible for fighting the unhealthy bacteria and fungi. The use of barrier methods like condoms for the male and the female should be freely recommended/advertised for prevention of STD's and HIV-AIDS.

In spite of all efforts if the tubes are blocked the couple can resort to advanced treatment namely-IVF (In Vitro Fertilization).

Ovulatory dysfunctions (PCOS-Polycystic Ovarian Syndrome):

Obesity and polycystic ovarian syndrome (PCOS) are closely associated. Women with PCOS are on an average more obese than their non PCOS counterparts with 50% having a body mass index (BMI) over 30 kg/m^3.Women with PCOS generally misinterpret this relationship, supposing that PCOS leads to obesity. The fact is that obesity drives polycystic ovaries to be more clinically manifest. Thus, obesity converts some women with occult polycystic ovary morphology to clinically obvious PCOS.Every physician treating women with PCOS has to become an expert in obesity management.

Preconceptional counseling in women with PCOS should identify risk factors for reproductive failure and correct them prior to treatment initiation. In this respect, it is imperative to recognize the presence of obesity and its centripetal distribution. Weight loss is recommended as first line therapy in obese women with PCOS seeking pregnancy. This recommendation is based on extrapolation from the benefits of weight loss seen in multiple other conditions, such as diabetes and cardiovascular disease, as well as recognition of obesity's association with poor reproductive outcome.

However, it should be noted that there is a paucity of studies suggesting that weight loss prior to conception improves live birth rate in obese women with or without PCOS (Moran et al., 2006) On the other hand, multiple observational studies have noted that weight loss is associated with improved spontaneous ovulation rates in women with PCOS (Pasquali et al., 2003; Moran et al 2006).In fact, pregnancies have been reported after losing as little as 5% of initial body weight.

Diet: It is generally agreed that energy restriction is required for weight loss. In fact, early improvements in reproductive function in the absence of apparent weight loss were probably due to energy restriction per se. However, there is little agreement on what constitutes the optimal diet for women with PCOS.

The resurgence of the Atkin's diet (Low carbohydrate diet) has generated considerable interest in very low calorie diets in recent years. This diet can lead to significantly decreased body weight in PCOS. With a shift in focus of treating doctors on hyperinsulinemia in cases of PCOS the components of diet that are most potent in stimulating insulin release have become a particular target for women with the syndrome. This includes removal of refined sugar and simple carbohydrates which are absorbed quickly and converted to glucose as measured by their glycemic index, (glucose is given the highest glycemic index). Carbohydrates with a low glycemic index usually have a high fiber content allowing glucose to be retained within the gut for slower release, leading to lower peak plasma glucose concentrations and therefore a lower insulin response. It is effective to reduce carbohydrate intake altogether to the point where the body begins to metabolize adipose tissue leading to ketogenesis (which can be measured in the urine). This process is the basis of the Atkin's diet.

The second issue is the timing of meals. The insulin release after a single large meal is greater than the accumulated insulin secretion from several small meals of equivalent calorie content. In addition, skipping meals may reduce metabolic rate slightly and commencing calorie intake early in the day appears to reduce later intake.

Exercise:

Insufficient physical activity might explain why women with PCOS have a tendency towards overweight/obesity. Baseline activity levels by self report were less in women with PCOS compared with control women (Wright et al 2004). It is clear that regular physical activity is an important component of weight loss programmes, because it is associated with better long term weight loss maintenance. Increased physical activity is recommended for obese women with PCOS. However, it is always advisable to consider the possible orthopaedic and cardiovascular limitations of the individual.

Vaginismus (fear of penetration):

Definition: Vaginismus is the involuntary spasm of the pelvic muscles surrounding the outer third of the vagina specifically the levator ani and perineal muscles severe enough to prevent vaginal penetration of the penis during sexual intercourse excluding the organic causes of dysparuenia (To summarize – it is the phobic anxiety to penetration).

Sexuality is a taboo in our society and the inhibitions attached to the topic of sex refrains the patients from seeking medical help. It has been estimated that nearly half the couples face some type of sexual dysfunction in their lifetime, which may be expressed in the form of lack of arousal, decreased libido, premature ejaculation, impotence, vagisnismus etc.

In a gynaecology clinic, patients often report with complaints of failure to consummate marriage. Some complain of dysparaneuia, i.e., painful intercourse. The added pressure of child bearing brings them to an infertility clinic. Therefore, there is a need to recognize and treat vaginismus with the techniques of sensate focus, which are very simple to practice.

Sensate Focus: In 1970 Masters & Johnson's described the technique called ' Sensate focus', which is a therapy used for sexual dysfunctions, designed to increase communication, strengthen relationships and experience sexual intercourse by focusing on the likes and dislikes of the partner. Kegel's exercises and stepwise learning of sexual intercourse are the added components.

A retrospective study was undertaken in a period of 3 years (2001-2003) to analyze the sociocultural and medical factors associated infertility with sensate focus. Of the total 2083 infertile patients, 17 reported with vaginismus, where the mean age of wife was 27 years (range 21-36 years) and the mean age of husband was 30.8 years (range 26-40 years).The mean duration of marriage was 4.2 months (24-97 months).

Desire for pregnancy was the predominant cause for reporting at the clinic in 10 women; 5 requested treatments for both infertility and resolution of the sexual problem and only 2 women wanted resolution for sexual problem first. Women with longer duration of marriage wanted treatment for infertility first.

Social pressure for pregnancy brought 8 couples to the clinic, marital disharmony was reported in 4 couples and 10 men complained of work pressure affecting the relations, which was an excuse to escape from the problem. Surprisingly, the incidence of love marriage was significantly high in this group (35.3%).

The severity of vaginismus as described by Lamont is given below, which is purely situational to intercourse or examination by a doctor.

Grade 1-Perineal and levator spasm (2 patients)

Grade 2-Perineal spasm maintained throughout pelvic Examination (4 patients).

Grade 3-Levator spasm and elevation of buttocks (4 patients)

Grade 5- Refusal to examination (1 patient)

Ovulation was present in 8 women, and was absent in 3 and not investigated in 6.

The clinicians' approach to treatment:

The first most important aspect of treatment is counseling of both partners by developing a comfortable dialogue between the therapist and the partners in complete privacy. The doctor should spend time in explaining the mechanism of the problem to the couple. This should include education of the couple on normal anatomy and physiology of reproductive system.

The woman should be explained the genesis of vaginismus showing her the related diagrams and explaining the way in which she is stopping penetration.

After 2-3 sessions, once the confidence in the therapist is gained, a brief history of the past experiences should be taken. Most of the patients express their hidden fears of physical or emotional child abuse. In the study mentioned above, one woman complained of beating by father and another reported alcoholism in father. One patient complained of incest and alcoholism in father.

For management of such cases, various tasks are assigned to both partners with the aim to eliminate anxiety of performance by forbidding intercourse initially. Non demanding tasks like pleasure giving mutual stimulation according to the likes and dislikes of the partner are explained to them with an aim to increase communication between the husband and wife. Genital stimulation is prohibited first. Then stepwise, they can proceed to genital stimulation, penetration and complete intercourse.

In severe cases of vaginismus, the female partners may be assisted with vaginal wall moulds or plastic dilators and taught self insertion with the help of Kegel's exercises.

After such regime the couples generally report with favorable results after 1-2 sittings. Further tasks are assigned to motivate both the partners.

In above study 10 couples had complete resolution and could resume active sexual intercourse. In two couples sexual relations did not improve despite the improvement in the female partner's ability to control vaginal muscles.

Two couples were referred to the psychiatrist due to secondary impotence in the male partner. Three couples were lost to follow up.

Pregnancy was achieved in 10 couples of which 6 (35.3%) were spontaneous conceptions, 3 required ovulation induction and intrauterine insemination due to ovulatory dysfunction and one conceived with IVF-ET.

This example was given here just to illustrate that much can be achieved in many cases of infertility without using any medicine or surgery.

References

1. Adam H Balen, Gerard S Conway, Roy Homburg, Richard S Legro A Guide to clinical management of PCOS.
2. Brinsden Peter: Textbook of In Vitro Fertilization and Assisted Reproduction 1.2; 11(p) 189-216.
3. Clayton RN, Ogden V, Hodgkinson J, Worswick et al. How common are polycystic ovaries in normal women and what is their significance for the fertility of the population?. Clin Endocrinol 1992;37:127-134.
4. Fordney DS, Dyspareunia and vaginismus Clinical Obstet. Gynaecol. 1978:21(1):205.
5. Franks S,Adams J, Mason HD, Polson DW.Ovulatory disorders in women with polycystic ovary syndrome.Cl;in Obstet Gynecol 1985;12:605-632.
6. Glueck CJ, Wang P, Goldenberg N, Siev-Smith L. Pregnancy outcomes among women with polycystic ovary syndrome treated with Metformin. Hum Reprod 2002 ; 17:2858-2864.

7. Human Reproduction 2008: 23 :(3):463-477, Consensus on infertility treatment related to polycystic ovarian syndrome.
8. Masters W, Johnson V-Human sexual inadequacy .Boston. Little Brown 1970.
9. Martin Weisberg; Physiology of female sexual function.
10. Moran C, Knochenhauer E, Boots LR, Azziz R. Adrenal androgen excess in hyperandrogenism;Relation to age and body mass.Fertil Steril1998; 71:671-674.
11. Rajan-Post graduate Reproductive endocrinology.
12. Ruutiainen K Erkkola R, Gronroos MA, Irjala K. Influence of body mass index and age on the grade of hair growth in hirsute women of reproductive ages.Fertil Steril 1998; 50:260-265.

22

Infertility Woes: Experiences of an Infertility Specialist

Nirmal Bhasin

Introduction:

The life style modifications of the 21st century have brought us to the threshold where we want everything at the click of a button according to our wishes and command at our convenient time. We try to control Nature and as a result distort our natural resources.

Many couples postpone having a family for various reasons like education, career, financial or social reasons and then suddenly they wake up to want a baby immediately. They seek help of doctors, astrologers, and friends and stress themselves out with repeated failures. The stress of infertility treatment adds on as they cannot cope with the demands of adequate and appropriate treatment for infertility. For example, very soon after starting the treatment they find that too much time is required to visit the clinics; the money spent on treatment also start looking exorbitant and the main problem is that they have to face the fact that the success rate of all such efforts is as low as 20-30 %.

Infertility treatment requires patience as well as proper understanding of the kind of cooperation needed from the couples. Hence, counseling is a key element in any infertility service. Counseling should be done by qualified, trained personnel. However, the treating doctors usually do not devote adequate time for counseling to both the partners.

Coping with failure is difficult for everybody- patients, treating doctors and counselors alike. All of them can be equally confused, angry, distressed, depressed and very often in tears because of the incidents of failure faced by them. Many a times, as a treating infertility specialist, I stop my tears from flowing in the presence of patients.

In this chapter I want to share some of my experiences in the past 9 years of my association with patients seeking help to conceive.

Case 1

At the age of 50 Surjit Kaur (name changed) had lost her 23 year old son in an accident 3 months ago. She came from UK with the hope to get her son back through IVF treatment. She was totally shattered after his death as she was now left with a daughter in law, her son's widow. I tried to convince her to abandon the idea of treatment at her age and with a daughter in law. But she was adamant and had the permission from her daughter in law to go ahead with the IVF.She was counseled for IVF with ovum donation and she readily agreed. A donor was selected and stimulated for the process, at the same time Surjit's womb was prepared to accept the embryos. On the day of oocyte retrieval 8 oocytes were retrieved of which 6 had fertilized. Four embryos were transferred into Surjit's uterus at 4 cell stage. Her faith was very strong and she stayed confined to bed for 15 days praying all the time. She was told to keep minimal activity but she wouldn't listen. ***"I have to prepare myself to welcome my son back".*** After 15 days she came with a positive report and had a picture of her son in her hands, which she showed to me saying ***"He's coming back to me".*** I was speechless; she did not have any tears or smiles-only a peaceful expression on her face. She delivered a healthy male child in UK with caesarean section and named him Manjit after her first son.

Case 2

It was 7 am and I was trying to gather courage to face Pooja (name changed) in her hospital room. The effect of sedatives given to her last night had weakened. She heard her mother crying helplessly. All she could recall was the series of events last night; she had called her gynecologist complaining of pain in the lower abdomen, her visit to the hospital, a check up, an ultrasound and deep sleep. She felt the emptiness in her belly and screamed ***"Where's my baby? Where's my baby!"*** Her cries mingled with her mother's synchronously.

Pooja a strong willed, optimistic and cheerful lady in her late twenties always brought smiles to our faces whenever she visited us at the fertility centre. She was battling with infertility for 8 years.

I had the opportunity to perform the first IVF procedure independently as an embryologist after an year long training in an IVF lab. The nervousness prevailed for more than a week; I had been revising every step in my mind repeatedly. The egg retrieval procedure was conducted smoothly. I managed to identify eight star like oocytes under the microscope. They were kept with the husband's sperms for fertilization in the incubator. After a sleepless night on the next day I peered under the microscope and I felt I had conquered the world. Seven beautiful zygotes were smiling at me, they grew further the next day and four of them were gently transferred into Pooja's womb. The 15 days wait was a long one for all of us. She came with a positive blood report for pregnancy and our clinic celebrated this achievement and I got a pat on my back from my boss.

Pooja's visit to the clinic for her regular check ups were cheerful and I shared a special bond with her.She was now 22 weeks pregnant.

Yesterday night she called her gynecologist in distress, she had severe pain in her lower abdomen. I rushed to the hospital to see her; she was sedated and had expelled the premature baby. I felt totally helpless & and I felt hollow in my heart. Today I was afraid to face her. As I entered her room she stopped crying, looked at me, smiled and said, ***"Thank you Doctor- at least I can be a mother"***.

Case 3

"I feel incomplete and have no desire to live" said Sujata 6 years ago. She was 35 years then, married to a businessman. She was suffering from endometriosis and had fibroids in her uterus. She had undergone 6 cycles of IVF at various centres in India. Every month she grieved and cried- ***"I feel useless and unwanted in this family"***. In addition to her psychological stress she had added pressure from her husband and mother in law. They wanted her husband to remarry and get an heir for the family. Her husband insisted her to stay with him and permit him to have a second wife. Sujata was a highly qualified professional and could not agree to his proposal. He started harassing and beating her frequently. Finally she divorced him, but life became from bad to worse. The loneliness was killing her- ***"At least I had a family"*** She would curse her destiny and weep silently.

Her friends and parents, with difficulty convinced her to remarry; she wouldn't agree blaming herself for not being able to mother a child. She finally agreed under the condition that all her problems would be disclosed to her perspective husband. Finally a good match, a widower with a 16 year old son was found for her. A low profile marriage was arranged with only the family members to bless the couple. Today Sujata is happily married for the last five years and is blessed with a son who loves her. ***He grew in her heart not in her womb.***

Conclusion:

One of the main purposes of this chapter is to guide those with experience in counseling methods to understand the clinical, scientific and emotional background of patients suffering from infertility. The paramedical staff, social worker, NGO's can all unite to help people overcome this emotional disorder. As infertility is a social problem also the social organizations are in a unique position to assist in the counseling role. The case reports are a medium to spread the message about the inner feelings and fears of the patients. They need to be listened to patiently, comforted and guided to the right doctor for treatment.

Reference

Case histories from day to day practice (1999 – 2008)

23

Management of Knee Joint Pain in Elderly by 'Application of Moist Heat'

Parminder Kaur, Indarjit Walia and Sushma Kumari Saini

Musculoskeletal pain is a major health problem among geriatric population. Most of geriatric population (45- 83%) is troubled by chronic pain in knee joint that have major effect on their quality of life. Due to continuous suffering and discomfort, functional capacity reduces which leads to cessation of activities at home, work and in leisure time. Under treated or poorly managed knee joint pain can affect their physical, psychological, social, and emotional life of the patients. These real life consequences of knee joint pain need to be given adequate attention in the home care settings.

The goal of treatment is **to minimize pain** and its impact on their quality of life. Different pain relief methods are often classified as pharmacological and non-pharmacological. Pharmacological (medicinal) treatment is associated with many side effects such as acidity, ulcer, bleeding etc. Moreover, medicines are very expensive. Non pharmacological methods of pain control i.e. exercise, rest and joint protection, heat and cold therapy, hydrotherapy, patient education, psychological support, weight control, exercise and heat application etc can also be used to relieve pain if practiced regularly and properly (alone or in combination with medicines. These practices have the added advantage that there is no risk of adverse drug interaction. One of such non-pharmacological approaches is the moist heat therapy.

Benefits of Moist Heat Therapy are as under:

- Moist heat is more effective than dry heat as it penetrates more than dry heat with the same temperature.
- It has additional capacity to change the tissue temperature rapidly and more vigorous response from temperature receptors.
- It increases the extensibility of collagen tissues.
- It decreases joint stiffness in tendons and ligaments.
- It relieves pain and muscle spasms.
- It increases blood flow and stimulates faster healing.
- It increases metabolic activity.

Moist Heat can be given in the form of hot pack, placed on painful area of the joint. An application for about 15 minutes will relieve the pain. A warm shower, hot moist towel or moist heating pad can also be used to provide moist heat.[36] Hot bath, steamed towels, hot compress therapy can also be used for application of moist heat to small areas of body. Hot compresses are notably effective for both mild and serious chronic muscle problems.

Moist Heat Application Procedure (Annexure-V)

Articles: Big Basin, Jug with hot water, Towels, Soap

Procedure:

- Collect all the articles at one place.
- Client should sit comfortably on a stool/chair/bed.
- Wash hands.
- Expose only the area to be treated.
- Assess the area for any redness and swelling before the intervention.
- Take hot water in the jug.
- Pour hot water into the basin, dip the towel, squeeze out extra water and shake it well for the steam to escape.
- Check the temperature by applying it on the back of your hand. Apply the moist hot towel over the knee joint and cover it with the dry towel/cloth.

- Change the moist hot towel every 4 to 5 minutes (four times).
- The procedure is to be continued for total duration of 20 minutes twice a day.
- Dry the area with the clean towel.
- Inspect the area for any redness or blisters.
- Replace the articles after washing.
- Wash hands with soap and water.

Evidence of efficacy of moist heat

A study was conducted in National Institute of Nursing education, PGIMER, Chandigarh on a sample of 43 patients in experimental group and 44 in control group. Intensity of knee joint pain was assessed with the visual analogue scale (a standardized scale). Moist heat was used as an intervention for knee joint pain. Subjects on pain killers were asked to continue if they feel the need of it. Moist heat was applied for 20 min twice a day among experimental group for seven days. No intervention was given among the control group. On the 8th day there was significant reduction in the intensity of pain in the right as well as the left knee in experimental group as compared to the control group. Intake of pain killer was decreased significantly in the experimental group as compared to control group after moist heat application. Therefore, from the study results it can be concluded that application of moist heat had a beneficial effect on knee joint pain.

References

1. Kenneth D. Community oriented program for the control of rheumatic diseases: Studies of rheumatic disease in the developing world. Journal of Current Opinion in Rheumatology 2005; 17(2): 153-156.
2. Martin U. Chronic knee pain in the elderly. 2005; 5: 1-10.
3. Walter L, Calmbach MD. Evaluation of patients presenting with knee pain. Journal of American Academy of Family Physicians 2003: 1-9.
4. Artificial joint. Total knee replacement [online] 2005: Available on http://www.artificialjoint.com/tkr/ arthritis/tkrtext.htm.
5. Falk KM. Pain management [online] 2005: http://www.nursece.com/online course/html/05.

6. McAlindon TE, Cooper C, Kirwan JR, Dieppe PA. Knee pain and disability in the community. British Journal Rhumatology 1992; 31(3): 189-92.
7. Anthony D, Bruce P. Burden of major musculoskeletal condition. Bulletin of the World Health Organization 2003; 81: 640-656.
8. Bhutia TK. A study to assess the health complaints and related self care ability among the geriatric population 1997: 5-6.
9. Ulf Jacobbson. Pain management among older people in need of help with activities of daily living. Journal of Pain Management Nurse 2004; 5(4): 137-143.
10. Baird CL. First line treatment poor oestioarthritis part 2. Non-pharmacologic interventions and evaluation. Journal of Orthopaedics Nurse 2001; 20(6):18-20.
11. Chung SC, Kim H.S. The effect of stabilization splint on the TMJ closed lock. Cranio 1991; 11(2):95-101.
12. Lehman JF. Therapeutic heat and cold. 4th ed. Williams and Willsins Baltimore.1982: 619-28.
13. Kozier B, Erb G, Blais K, Wilkinson JM . Fundamentals of nursing concepts process and practice. 5th ed. California: Addition Wesley Nursing 1995: 1386-87.
14. Hot Application. The analyst – internet health report: treatment: hot applications [online] 2005: http://www.digitalnaturopath.com / treat/T324897. html.
15. Kaur P, Walia IJ and Saini SK. A quasi experimental study on effectiveness of moist heat application on knee joint pain in Daddu Majra Colony, Chandigarh. An unpublished thesis of National Institute of Nursing Education, PGIMER, Chandigarh submitted to Punjab University Chandigarh, 2007.

24

Managing Severe Malnutrition without Any Hospitalization/ Medicine

Santosh Kumari, Tanzin Dikid, Sitanshu Shekhar Kar and AJ Singh

Even 40 years after green revolution, India still faces the problem of malnutrition. The third National Family Health Survey (NFHS-3) concluded that almost half of children under five years of age (48 percent) are stunted and 43 % are underweight. The proportion of children who are severely undernourished is also notable: 24 percent are severely stunted and 16 percent are severely underweight.

In view of the high prevalence of malnutrition in India, the government had launched several nutritional programmes at the national level, like special nutritional program, mid day meal scheme, applied nutrition program and integrated child development services (ICDS) scheme. Similarly, many nutrition intervention programs are being implemented in many developing countries with varying success rates.

The mass approach inherent in any such program is more or less impersonal. Such approach does not involve the family intimately. It has also been observed that the functionaries of these programs often take the intervention casually. Their focus remains mainly on the management and accounting of supplies and on maintenance of records. The individual beneficiary of the program, i.e., the child, usually remains ignored and neglected. And many times severely malnourished children continue to deteriorate despite the program. It has also been reported that Anganwadi workers are often asked by their superiors to not to register severe malnutrition cases in their records. Apparently, this is done to improve the record/report of the centre/department. This paradox implies that the program, by and large, caters to relatively better off children while grade 3 and 4 children who should be the prime focus of the program, are not at all benefited by the programme.

As a contrast, if parents are instructed about nutritional care of the malnourished child on individual level and a regular follow up is done, constant improvement in the condition of the child can be achieved.

Guidelines for management of malnutrition state that provision of inpatient treatment is the only way to treat severely malnourished children. However, in resource constrained settings such as ours it puts considerable strain on our already crowded health infrastructure. Admission to the hospital requires the care givers (most often parents) to leave their work, leading to loss in terms of productive capacity and entails loss in terms of opportunity costs.

On the other hand, research has shown that domiciliary treatment of severe malnutrition is more cost effective and shows promising results. In Bangladesh, the recovery rate of severely malnourished children treated with 1 week's inpatient care followed by home management was similar to that of children in a specialized nutrition unit. Home based treatment was more than four times cheaper than centre based care, and was preferred by mothers. As an example, consider Rinku's story (name changed).

Rinku was born on 16th January 1999 at home in a resettlement colony to a primipara mother in a joint family. Both parents were educated up to tenth standard. The family owned a small tea shop. His mother got married at 19 years of age. His birth weight was 1600 grams. Breastfeeding was initiated on third day of life, but was discontinued at one month of age. His maternal as well as paternal grand-mother instructed his mother to stop breast feeding him as her milk was not considered to be healthy for the child.

There is a belief in north India that in some women the breastmilk is "not good" for babies. This kind of diagnosis is usually made by elder ladies in the household when a child is not able to gain weight with breast feeds. In fact, an 'ant test' is popular in villages. In this test, mother's milk is expressed in a cup and an ant is put in it. If the ant dies the mother's milk is declared as 'not good' for the baby.

In Rinku's case also mother's milk was not considered good for him. He was given bottle-feeds with half strength milk. Bottle was boiled once daily.

Contact with State health care service/ICDS: Mother and child were not registered with *anganwari* as his mother had come to visit her parents to assist in the delivery of her sister-in-law.

In the month of November (age-10 months) his mother came to our dispensary to enquire about measles vaccine. At that time child had upper respiratory infection .On examination his weight was 3.75 kilogram, hairs were thin and easily pluckable, cheeks bony, no teeth had erupted, he could neither sit nor crawl. On auscultation, chest had crepts. He was irritable. His mother told that he did not have a sound sleep during night. His diet was deficient in calories and iron. He was referred to the local dispensary where he was prescribed medicines for infection.

When enquired from his mother why he was not given any supplementary feed, she told he had "*Soka / Parchhanwa*". He did not accept any feed and vomited it out. He was too weak to tolerate supplementary feeds. The family had spent more than 2000 rupees on his treatment without any result, and they felt that he would never recover.

It was then that a home visit was paid by a nurse (Mrs Santosh) to train the mother in steam inhalation. Dietary advice was also given. Second home visit was paid next day to assess his condition. He had improvement in his respiratory problem. He was being given bottle feed. However, the bottle was visibly very dirty. Mother was told to stop bottle-feeding. Hazards of bottle feeding were explained to her. A menu (diet plan) was prepared for the child. The mother was demonstrated how to prepare *sujee kheer*, mashed banana etc. Spoon feeding was started. Initially he resisted, but later on he enjoyed the feed. The mother was told not to add water in milk. She was also told to feed him every 2-3 hours.

Third home visit was paid after four days. The mother was happy with the progress of her child. She told that he was better; accepting feeds and slept well during night. After one week his weight was 4 kilograms. The mother was encouraged to continue feeding as instructed. After one month of intervention weight was taken again, it was 5 kilograms. He could sit, and asked for things with gestures. After two months of our intervention, he started crawling, and weight gain continued. After three months his weight was six kilograms, i.e. he shifted to grade 2 malnutrition from grade 4, had 4 teeth and he started standing with support. His mother was motivated to continue feeding him and increase the diet with home cooked food. She was also asked to visit *anganwadi*. His grandmother was also very happy that child had improved without any medication.

But after that the mother went back to her in-law's place. Her mother in law was happy to see the health of the child. She said "it is surprising that the child had improved without any medication and without spending any money." At her in law's place she got busy with her routine work and could not take care of her son properly. She came to Chandigarh again for follow-up after three months. The weight gain had stopped and she had started bottle feeds again. Again, she was motivated to continue feeding as advised earlier. She was asked to come for follow-up again after one month. Thereafter the child started improving. He also gained weight. He started walking. After that there was no follow up for sometime.

At present, he is 9 years old and studying in fourth standard, his growth is like any other child of his age. His weight is 30 kilograms.

A similar case of a female child Shivani was managed at community level by one of the authors (SSK). Essentially, she was a grade IV malnutrition case. Her weight was only 5.5 kg at the age of 1 year11 months when she was brought to our health centre by her mother with complaints of repeated episodes of diarrhea. She was listless with delayed milestones (not able to stand etc).Only breastfeeding was being given. Her calorie intake was only 500 per day. Proper counseling of the mother was done. Feeding was explained. She was regularly followed up by our team. Eventually, she gained weight steadily and shifted to grade II malnutrition within 3 months. No hospitalization was required.

A third case report, described hereunder shares our experience of home based management of a case of severe malnutrition during the posting of principal investigator (TD) in a rural health training centre of PGIMER in district Ambala, in the North Indian state of Haryana.

During a routine anganwadi (day care centre) health check-up of under five year children in March 2008, we came across a girl child Neha, 7 month 28 days old suffering from loose stools. On clinical examination, the child was lethargic with some signs of dehydration with delayed milestones with PEM grade IV with milestones corresponding to 3 months of age. She did not have any oedema.

Neha belonged to a poor family with four family members where the father was a daily wager and the only breadwinner for the family. When the birth history of the mother was elicited, it was found that she was the second child of the couple, the first child (also a female) had expired at around 7 months of age due to pneumonia. Both the children were delivered at home. On inquiring about the diet history of the child it was found that she was inadequately weaned and was being fed tea. Each child (0-5yrs) in the catchment area is registered in the anganwadi and monitored for growth and provided supplementary nutrition along with informal education. While Neha's name was registered in the anganwadi centre (AWC), she had not received any supplementary nutrition so far.

The child was given ORS for diarrhoea, the mother and the grandmother of the child were told about the child's condition and prognosis explained to them. They were advised to take the child to nearest health care facility for admission and management of grade IV PEM. But the family expressed their inability in taking the child to a hospital as they did not have adequate financial resources. Clearly, Neha was fighting a loosing battle.

The turnaround:

The RHTC team took it upon themselves to manage the child in the existing resources. A team was made in the village comprising of various stakeholders such as RCH/ ICDS/ women's committee such as *mahila mandal* and *sakshar mahila samuh*. The team informed the community development project officer (CDPO) about the non-receipt of nutritional supplement by the child. A supervisor was sent to the village in the ensuing week to look into the matter and supply of supplementary food for the child was ensured. The food was rationed to the baby on a weekly basis. Weekly visits were paid to the family by the RHTC team. The family was instructed by the team at frequent intervals on topics relevant to infant feeding, disease prevention, family planning and use of easily available ingredients to prepare nutritious meals for the child. The child was given an oral dose of vitamin A (1 lakh IU), an oral dose of albendazole (200ml). In between, the child again developed diarrhoea for which she was given ORS powder and zinc supplementation from the local sub-centre and monitored for signs of dehydration. Weight of the child was monitored during these weekly visits. The median rate of weight gain was approx. 19gm/ day. Her milestones started to improve. She started sitting with support 40 days into the therapy. Within four months she has shifted from grade IV malnutrition to grade II.

Conclusion:

Domiciliary treatment of severe malnutrition with close supervision as an integrated public health response model is feasible as the present case studies show. It involves community consultation, mobilization and participation with due consideration of factors such as socioeconomic condition of the family, high workload for women, less desirability of a daughter, illiteracy and underutilization of available health and nutritional supplementation services. At home care is less disruptive to domestic routines and allows mothers to continue with house work and other family responsibilities and is therefore associated with low opportunity costs to the family. It also avoids a situation of congregation of children to a hospital or day care centre thus avoiding exposure to acquired infections.

These case studies show that even severely malnourished children can be managed at home. They just need constant follow up and counseling regarding nutrition. This can easily be done by a paramedical worker /nurse at primary care set up. Success can thus be attained by personal attention and care rather than hospitalization or medication.

References

1. International Institute of Population Sciences (IIPS) and ORC Macro. National Family Health Survey (NFHS-3), 2005-06. Mumbai: IIPS, 2007.
2. Boelaert M, Davis A, Le Lin B et al. Nutrition guidelies (1st edn). Paris: Medecins sans Frontieres, 1995.
3. Ville de Goyet C, Seaman J, Geijer U. The management of nutriotionalemergencies in large populations. Geneva: WHO, 1978.
4. WHO, UN High Commissioner for Refugees (UNHCR), World Food Programme (WFP), International federation of red cross and red crescent societies (IFRC). The management of nutrition in major emergencies. Geneva, 1998.
5. Khanum S, Ashworth A, Huttley S R. Controlled trial of three approaches to the treatment of severe malnutrition. *Lancet* 1994; 344: 1728-32.
6. Ashworth A, Khanum S. Cost effective treatment for severely malnourished children: what is the best approach? *Health Policy Plan* 1997; 12: 115-21.
7. Collins S, Sadler K. Outpatient care for severely malnourished children in emergency relief programmes: a retrospective cohort study. *Lancet* 2002; 360: 1824-30.

Fig. 1

Sequence of events that led to detection of PEM grade IV in the community and subsequent intervention (Neha's case study)

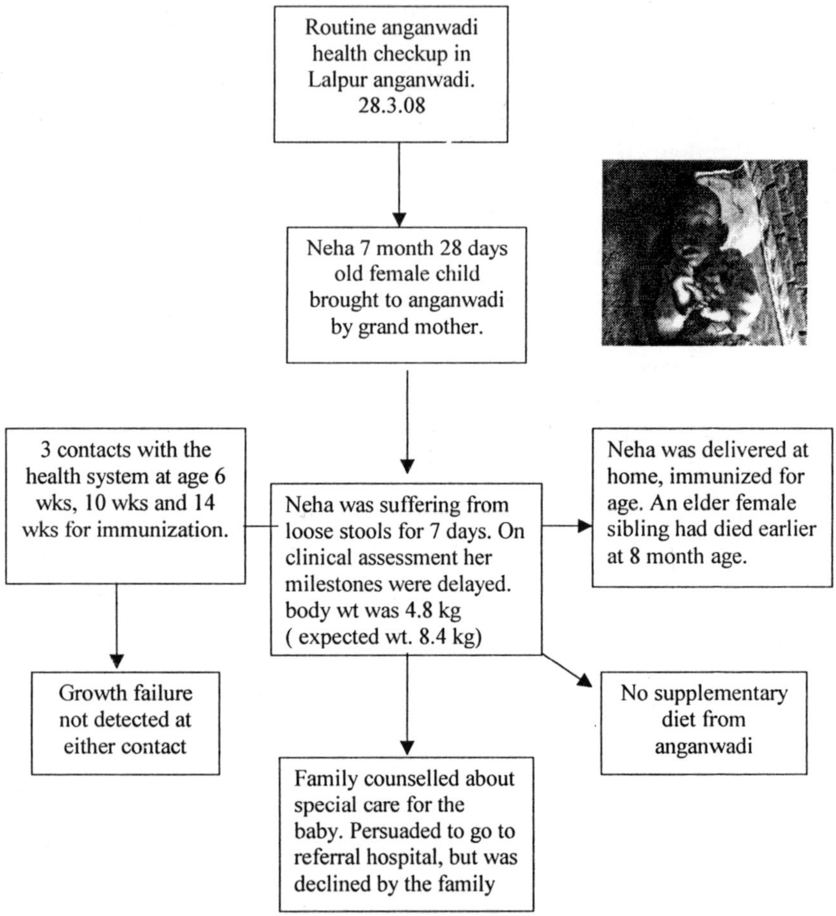

Fig. 2
Community based management model evolved

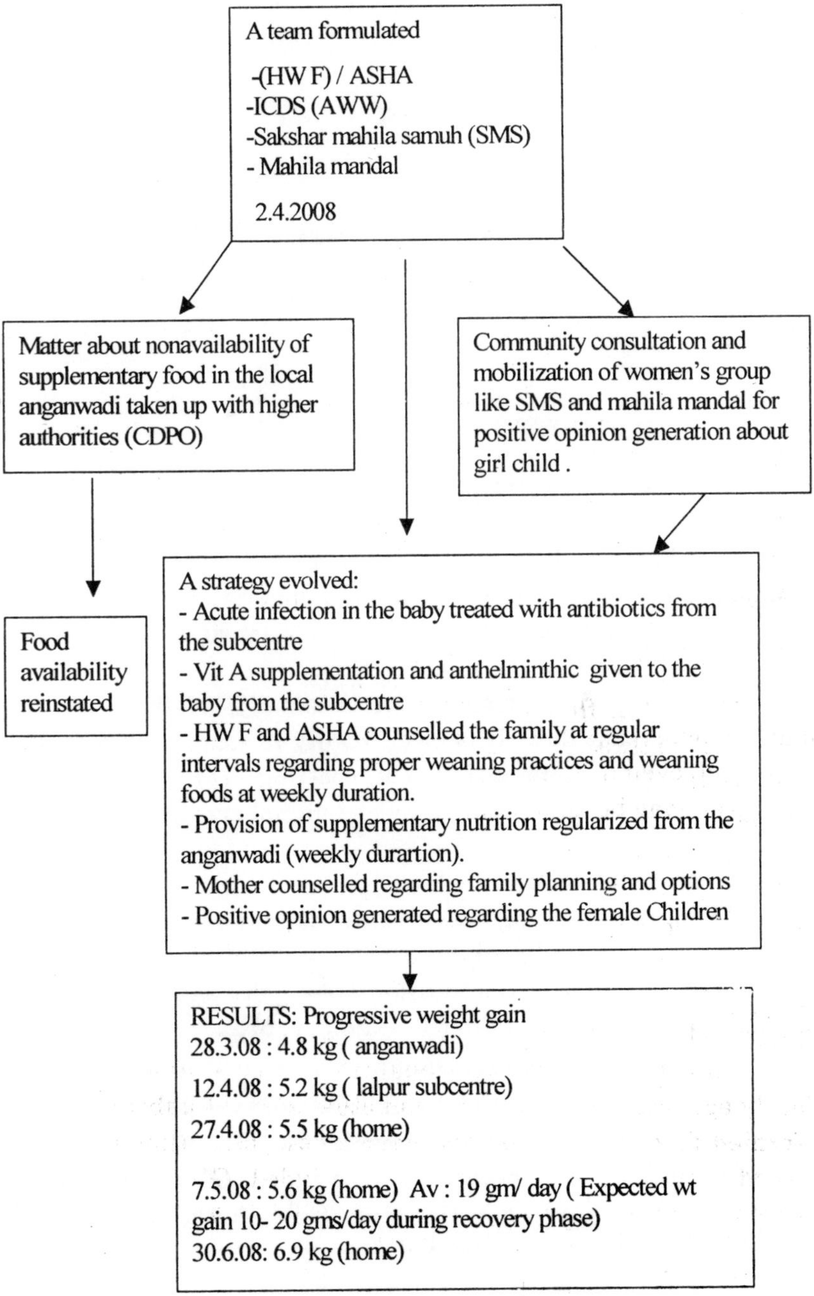

25

Menarche

Meera Dhuria, Suneela Garg and VK Gupta

Menarche is an important landmark in the life of woman. It is the first menstrual period, which typically occurs about 2 years after thelarche. From both social and medical perspectives it is often considered the central event of female puberty, as it signals the possibility of fertility. It is the culmination of a series of physiological and anatomic processes of puberty.

The initial flow of menarche is usually brighter red than mature menstrual flow. It is often scanty in amount and may be very brief, even a single instance of "spotting." Like other menses, menarche may be accompanied by abdominal cramping.

Medical Aspects of Menarche

When menarche occurs, it confirms that the girl has had a gradual oestrogen-induced growth of the uterus, especially the endometrium, and that the "outflow tract" (the passage) from the uterus, through the cervix to the vagina, is open.

In very rare instances, menarche may occur at an unusually early age, preceding thelarche and other signs of puberty. This is termed ***isolated premature menarche***, but other causes of bleeding must be investigated and excluded. Growth is usually normal. Isolated premature menarche is rarely the first manifestation of precocious puberty.

When menarche has failed to occur for more than 3 years after thelarche, or beyond 16 years of age, the delay is referred to as ***primary amenorrhea***.

Cultural aspects of menarche

Menarche is celebrated in many cultures around the world as rites of passage, a time to recognize that a girl is moving into womanhood. However, in majority of Indian states it is associated with sense of impurity. The compounding issues are reluctant mothers and teachers who fail to impart correct knowledge regarding menstruation.

TIMING OF MENARCHE:

The average age of menarche in various populations surveyed in the last several decades has ranged from 12.0 to 18.5 years. The earliest mean is reported for African-American girls and the oldest for high altitude subsistence populations in Asia.

FACTORS THAT CAN AFFECT THE TIMING OF MENARCHE

- Genetic factors
- Environmental factors especially family
- Nutritional status
- Physical activity and exercise
- Physical illness
- Stress and social factors

PROBLEMS ASSOCIATED WITH MENARCHE

- Isolated premature menarche
- Primary amenorrhea.
- Anovulatory cycles
- Dysmenorrhoea
- Social issues

NON MEDICAL/ NON MEDICINAL TREATMENT FOR THE PROBLEMS

Premature menarche

If the periods appear early than the usual age in a girl, following approach may be adopted.

- Reassurance
- Look for genetic association: The genetic association of timing is strongest between mothers and daughters. There will be a history that this thing runs in the family and that the mother of the girl also had her periods early.
- Often it is linked to obesity.Counseling for excessive weight gain may be tried, because, surplus calories (beyond growth and activity requirements) are reflected in the amount of body fat, which signals to the brain the availability of resources for initiation of puberty and fertility.
- Removal of conflict in the family relationships may also help since, psychological factors are also involved in early menarche.

Late menarche

Similarly, for girls who have their first period delayed beyond the usual age following regime may be tried.

- Reassurance
- Counsel for increased protein intake as lower protein intakes and higher plant fiber intakes are associated with later onset and slower progression of female puberty, i.e., such things are more seen in thinner girls!
- Increase calcium intake (milk and milk products) should be tried, as calcium deficiency can lead to delayed puberty.
- Increase exposure to sunlight
- Modulation of Physical activity: A high level of exercise, whether for athletic or body image purposes, or for daily subsistence, reduces energy calories available for reproduction and slows puberty. So in athletic girls periods may be delayed.
- Underlying disease may also be a cause of delayed periods. So, assess for any physical illness or chronic illness (TB) that may interfere with nutrition.
- Stress and social factors should also be taken in to consideration as psychological etiology may be there.
- Warmer, more supportive, low-stress family environment may help the girls in having their periods on usual time.

Dysmenorrhoea

In girls, who have painful periods, following measures may be undertaken.

*Reassurance
*Increase intake of Iron/ calcium rich diet
*Hot bath/ hot water bags
*Regular exercise

Anovulatory cycles

Many girls have periods without shedding of eggs. These are called as anovulatory cycles. In such cases increase in intake of iron rich diet may be tried.

In the problems listed above consultation with a doctor (or intake of medicine)may be required if abovementioned measures do not provide relief.

References

www.wikipedia.org.access on 6.04.08

www.webmed.com on 7.04.08.

Joan C Chrisler. From Menarche to Menopause: The female body in feminist therapy; 2004. Haworth Book Publication.

Acharya A, Reddaiah VP, Baridalyne N.Nutritional Status and Menarche in Adolescent Girls in an Urban Resettlement Colony of South Delhi.? IJCM Journal Vol. 31; No. 4: 2006-10 - 2006-12)

26

Menopause and HRT

AJ Singh and Sukhwinder Kaur

The word **menopause** literally means the permanent physiological, or natural, stoppage of menstrual cycles, from the Greek roots 'meno' (month) and 'pausis' (a pause, a cessation).The word is commonly used in regard to cessation of menses in human females, where menopause happens more or less in midlife, signaling the end of the fertile phase of a woman's life. The normal menopausal age range is 45 to 55 years[1].

Menopause starts as the ovaries begin to fail to produce an egg every month, this in turn interrupts the regular pattern of the hormone cycles. It gradually leads to the somewhat chaotic and long-drawn out shutting down of the whole reproductive system. As the body struggles to adapt to the rapidly changing levels of natural hormones, a number of symptoms appear eg lack of energy, hot flashes, palpitations, depression, anxiety, irritability, mood swings, lack of concentration, vaginal dryness and urgency of urination.

In Western countries these symptoms have been projected as a hormone deficiency syndrome i.e. menopause. As a consequence, **Hormone Replacement Therapy (HRT)** was evolved and vigorously promoted by various pharmaceutical companies all over the world to "replace" women's depleting hormone levels due to menopause and to relieve associated symptoms[2]. In contrast, women in countries like India, view menopause rather positively and take menopausal symptoms in their stride. Use of HRT is almost nil in rural India and is negligible in urban India. Reason for such differential use of HRT is due to the difference in the way menopause is viewed in the two settings. In youth-oriented Western cultures, menopause is frequently intertwined with fears of aging, loss of status and loss of sexuality. However, women have been reported to welcome menopause in developing countries like India[3-5], Thailand, Zimbabwe and Israel [6-8] and in some developed countries also [9,10].

Across the globe, women are divided in their views on menopause. Some take it as a medical condition requiring treatment, whereas others see it as a natural transition to be managed by natural means. Studies done by the authors have revealed that, by and large, menopause is viewed positively by women in north India. Moreover, the Indian women are socialized into a 'culture of silence' regarding various reproductive health problems experienced by them. At menopause, even if they experience some symptoms, they tend to ignore these and tolerate them silently. Instead, they give more value to the attainment of freedom from menses. So much so that in our studies some of them exclaimed that they had attained heaven. Many said, 'I have become a man now'. This statement reinforces the notion that the social status of women in India is very low. Attainment of 'manhood' at menopause is valued by them[3-5].

Elaborate rules of conduct and rituals associated with menstruation have been prescribed for women in India since antiquity. Women have been indoctrinated into leading a restrained and disciplined life during menstruation, from adolescence to middle age. Once this restriction of menstruation is over, it is natural that they feel immensely relieved at menopause. They become free from the burden of child-birth and from cultural restrictions imposed on the social and religious lives of women are said to relish the renewed freedom and influence in their families and communities that come with menopause.

The powerful postmenopausal Indian mother-in-law playing the role of matriarch to a large extended family of sons, sons' wives and grandchildren is a familiar image in India. Such a woman ideally enjoys respect, deference and unquestioned authority over others in her family – male as well as female. Freed from heavy work burdens and from the need to conform to strict standards of female modesty, she is able to move about outside the confines of her home, not only in order to carry out certain necessary tasks for the benefit of her household, but also to engage in social and religious activities that interest her. Within the home, the position of middle-aged wife and mother of sons is typically one of considerable security, ease and comfort, relative to that which she occupied at a younger age and relative to that of younger women within her own household. The middle-aged woman's needs and desires are likely to be well attended to and accorded some priority by other members of the family[4].

Furthermore, at this stage of life, a woman is capable of acting independently with respect to many areas affecting her own well-being in a way that the young daughter-in-law in such a family is not. The fact that the middle aged woman (whether in an extended or nuclear family) generally controls intra-household food distribution and the allocation of many other domestic resources places her in a favourable position to obtain at least her fair share of the family's resources in terms of nutrition, clothing and medical care, which she might not have been able to do as a junior woman in the household of her husband's parents[4]. Flint and colleagues also reported that, among the Rajputs of Northern India, women who no longer menstruate may emerge from 'purdah' and move around freely within their village[5]. Such a scenario is responsible for the positive view of menopause exhibited by postmenopausal women of India.

In a study conducted in north India by the authors also, the majority of women welcomed the attainment of menopause. They considered themselves cleaner after menopause, being relieved off the filth associated with menstruation. More than one-third women reported that they undertook additional/extra activities after attaining menopause – as they were free of various restrictions on account of the sense of cleanlines associated with menstruation; and they could freely visit temples, relatives and friends.

In Sub-Saharan Africa also, the postmenopausal years are viewed positively as a time when women gain respect in their families and communities. However, the perception of menopause in youth-oriented countries of developed countries is frequently intertwined with fears of aging, loss of status and loss of sexuality. As a consequence menopause has been thoroughly medicalized in western countries.

In most societies, menopause marks a turning point in a woman's life. After menopause, many restrictions on women's activities are lifted to permit their greater participation in public life and access to a wide range of occupations. So long as a woman is subject to menstrual cycles, her activities are circumscribed by religious taboos. Opportunities to develop their talents or to follow their particular interests are often denied to younger women who are supposed to look after the household and younger children. Once past child-bearing age, they are free of these restrictions[1]. This is particularly true for developing countries like India. In western countries, on the other hand, there are no such restrictions on the lives of women during their reproductive years. The focus on individualism encourages women to get 'maximum' out of their lives. When they reach middle age they vigorously try to retain their 'womanhood' and youth by resorting to HRT.

Thus, the implications of reaching menopause vary from one society to another depending on the political and economic structure of each society and the condition of life it provides for women of all ages, including their access to health care. The psychological reaction of women to menopause reflects the value system of the society and the social status assigned by it to the aging woman[2].

Thus, we have two contrasting approaches to menopause. The Western approach advocates HRT use. The Indian approach is essentially non medicinal.

In fact, after mid 1970s when international menopausal societies were formed in many countries quite enthusiastic pharmaceutical response was witnessed with flourishing of multibillion dollar HRT business. Everyone advocated HRT as the only solution to problem of menopause. Various advantages had also been linked with HRT use. Past research has shown that HRT may also help prevent osteoporosis, heart disease, short-term memory loss, depression, and other diseases in post-menopausal women.

However, over a period of time a lot of problems have been attributed to HRT use. Recent research has found that HRT may not provide these benefits and rather may pose other risks, most notably an increased risk of breast cancer and ovarian/endometrial cancer. In view of the controversies linked to HRT the Million Women Study was conducted. The study confirmed the fears of malignancy risks of HRT.

Armed with this new information, many medical experts and women are trying to weigh the true benefits and risks of HRT. Undoubtedly, HRT is the most effective way to treat hot flashes and other bothersome, sometimes debilitating, symptoms of menopause. However, research continues to show a link between HRT and an increased risk of breast cancer.

Eleventh and twelfth World Congress on Menopause held at Buneos Aires (2005) Madrid (2008) respectively have reflected that the focus is now shifting from 'hot flush' to highlight other 'advantages' of HRT viz sexuality and quality of life. This seems to be a countermove to divert the attention of the potential HRT users from MWS study results and to explore new ways of boosting the sagging HRT sales.

The radical shift in approach of IMS was clearly visible in 12th World Congress on Menopause after publication of MWS/HERS/WHI and other related studies. The dwindling interest of pharmaceutical companies was even more apparent as compared to 11th Congress at Argentina. While Yokohama and Berlin conferences had a big crowd (both of delegates and the sponsors), the Buneos Aires conferences had lesser attendance and the Madrid conference had least presence of clients (delegates). Stalls and exhibits by sponsors were lusterless and the enthusiasm of the company representatives was missing. Poster session had lesser number of displays and was given less importance.

In a subtle and clever way the focus of company sponsored studies on menopause seems to have shifted to issues other than vasomotor symptoms (hot flushes etc) and osteoporosis. Now they are focusing on HRTs benefit in improving sexuality and overall quality of life of women.

The stakeholders have honestly now admitted in a book entitled "Health Plan for the Adult Woman" that the general public is becoming increasingly aware that menopause (and its associated symptoms) is a normal life event and that many women were, therefore, resistant to its medicalisation.

Now this was an HONEST CONFESSION.

This book (sponsored by Novo Nodisk, Wyeth, Schering, Procter and Gamble) was provided to the delegates in the congress at Madrid in 2008, free of cost.

However, simultaneously they have cleverly attempted to widen the scope of medicalizing the life of women. They assert that most of the disorders e.g. osteoporosis (which were earlier said to be heralded by menopause) develops well in advance of menopause .....even in utero.....and that many women already have latent disease (i.e. before menopause) warranting secondary prevention. Through this statement they mean to say that, so far, whatever was being done for menopausal symptoms (read HRT), was an approach of secondary prevention i.e. after the disease has developed.

They exhort now that true PRIMARY PREVENTION is a premenopausal requirement best achieved by healthy lifestyle, good nutrition and exercise, This, they say, is ideal in most societies requiring little or no specific drug therapy or diagnostic testing. Unfortunately, these measures are very difficulty to enforce in adolescence and young adult who regard menopause a distant future event.

Moreover, the book admitted now that biological responses to menopause may differ in different societies and that relevance of medical literature based on studies of western women (The book severely criticized relative risk data of MWS?!!?) to the management of women of other ethnic background was questionable and needed to be culturally re-examined. The book recommends that the health care (and treatment plan) should be individualized and management should be adjusted according to the health status of women. For this, the book says, technology, though costly, is the answer.

Public Health Implications: impact of The Million Women Study

These results from the Million Women Study, together with the Women's Health Initiative trial from the USA, have influenced the use of HRT all over the world.

Because of such evidence, which had a potential to damage the HRT business, the Million Women Study was

commented upon by many experts who tried to defend the HRT by finding loopholes in the methodology adopted by the study.

However, despite such attempts by some experts to salvage the reputation of HRT the damage has already been done to the HRT market. Sales are already down. Interestingly, the HRT menopause clinic, which had been functioning in Nehru Hospital, PGIMER, Chandigarh is now more or less closed down with not many takers for HRT. And closure of a menopause clinic in an apex medical institute is an important signal which can not be ignored. So, as of now,

HRT is out of favor and out of fashion in India.

Besides the risks associated with HRT use, there are other hassles also associated with HRT use viz.

(i) It is costly. On a moderate estimate @ Rs.500/- per month x 12 months x 5 years Rs.30000/-will be spent during 5 years HRT regime for a woman

(ii) One needs to remember to take a pill daily

(iii) Before starting HRT, baseline investigations are required eg blood test, x-ray, pap smear etc.

(iv) Periodic check ups are also needed. There are also problems like break through bleeding.

(v) All this may further increase the expenditure and the botheration for the HRT users.

Also the issue pertaining to the duration for which HRT should continue also needs to be settled.

Many alternative medicine therapy trials for menopausal symptoms are also being tried nowadays. Various home remedies for menopausal symptoms practiced across the globe also need to be evaluated.

So, as of now, HRT use for menopausal symptoms, at best, be avoided. Symptomatic treatment may, of course, be tried. In fact, the Indian Menopause Society has started including advertisement of soy products on its back cover pages ....which quotes HRT as potentially harmful and expensive. It shows HRT to have adverse effect on cognition, to have side effect of vaginal bleeding and its carry a risk of breast and endometrial cancer, and not to be recommended for long term therapy.

References

1. Twiss JJ, Wegner J, Hunter M, Kelsay M, Rathe-Hart M, Salado W (2007). "Perimenopausal symptoms, quality of life, and health behaviors in users and nonusers of hormone therapy". *J Am Acad Nurse Pract* 19 (11): 602-13.
2. Singh A and Arora A.K.. Profile of menopausal women in rural north India, Climacteric 2005; 8:177-184.
3. Kaur S, Walia I, and Singh A. How menopause affects the lives of women in suburban Chandigarh, India, Climacteric 2004; 7:175-180.
4. Million Women Study Collaborators. Breast cancer and hormone-replacement therapy in the Million Women Study. Lancet 2003; 362:419-27.
5. Anonymous. Directory 2007-2008 Indian Menopause Society (Back inside Cover).
6. Birkhauser MH, Barbw DH, Notelovitz M, Rees CM (Eds), Management Handbook – Health Plan for the Adult Woman. London, Taylor and Francis, 2005.
7. Singh AJ, Kaur S and Walia I (2002) A Historical Perspective on Menopause and Menopausal Age. Bull. Ind. Inst. Med. 32, 121-135.
8. Kaur S, Walia I, Singh AJ (2004) Age at menopause and its correlation with different variables, Nursing and Midwifery Research Journal Vol. 1, No.1, 9-13.

27

Menstrual Problems of Adolescent Girls

Panna Lal and Dipanweeta Routray

INTRODUCTION

Adolescence is the transitional period linking childhood to adulthood. It involves physical, biological, and psychological changes in a girl at puberty. Age of adolescents is considered to be ranging from 10-19 years. The major stages of pubertal changes involves the physical growth, development of secondary sex organs and breasts, pubic and axillary hair growth, development of ovaries and genital organs, growth spurt and menstruation.

Menstruation is a normal part of women's reproductive life. To understand how it occurs one has to have knowledge about the various reproductive organs of female. In addition to the external organs viz vulva, a pair of labia majora and labia minora, and a clitoris, a woman has internal organs which include a pair of ovaries (producing egg) a uterus (the sac for the baby to grow), fallopian tubes connecting the ovaries to the uterus and a hollow tubular structure called vagina for sexual intercourse.

Menarche is the first menstruation in a female which occurs usually around 12 to 16 years in Indian girls. Often it comes as a surprise for the adolescent girls. Sometimes, it creates apprehension if the girl is not properly informed about it well in advance. However, one should not worry too much about it because it is a normal phenomenon.

NORMAL PHYSIOLOGY OF MENSTRUATION:

Once the menstruation starts, it is repeated every month. In the midcycle ovaries release an egg. It also releases a hormone (chemical regulator) called estrogen, which stimulates the growth of the lining of the uterus and another hormone called progesterone to prepare a suitable environment in the lining of the uterus to receive the fertilized egg. If the egg doesn't get fertilized by a sperm, the uterus sheds its lining resulting in menstrual flow every month. This flow repeats itself in a cycle of approximately 28 days. The duration of flow usually remains between 3-5 days and the estimated blood loss during one menstrual period is 50- 200 ml.[1] A deviation of 2 or 3 days from normal 28 days rhythm is quite common.

ABNORMAL MENSTRUATION:

Any abnormality in the amount of blood loss or in the interval of having menses or duration of flow is considered undesirable. The main problems associated with abnormal menstruation include: dysmenorrhea or painful periods, menorrhagia (excessive amount of bleeding), amenorrhea (lack of periods), premenstrual symptoms (PMS), and irregular menses.

Dysmenorrhea : A slight discomfort with menses is a normal phenomenon. But different studies in India suggest that painful bleeding is the most common problem associated with menses affecting nearly 50 % girls.[2] It is generally of two types (a) congestive pain- in this a woman experiences dull aching pain. It starts approximately one week before the menses and lasts through out. (b) spasmodic pain- during this a woman gets cramps which start just prior to menses and stop within 1-2 days of bleeding. Spasmodic pain is more common and approximately 67.0% of the girls suffer from this.[3] Simple pain killers (Mefenamic acid tablets) can relieve the pain. Here, it should be remembered that such medication should be taken before the discomfort starts. Otherwise the tablets may be vomited out i.e. girls should anticipate the time of onset of abdominal discomfort. Hot water bottle may also be equally effective. However, it is better to consult a doctor before a girl starts using these. If the daily activities get hampered due to pain or nausea (feeling of vomiting), the woman or girl should consult a doctor.

Menorrhagia: If there is any increase in amount of menstrual blood or duration of bleeding or both the condition is called menorrhagia. Increase in amount of blood flow means woman has to use twice the number of pads she was using in the previous cycles or bleeding is associated with clots. Usually, a woman needs three fully soaked pads per day during the regular cycles. If the duration of the cycle is more than seven days it is considered a long cycle. It is usually associated with dysmenorrhea or painful bleeding. It can be due to hormonal imbalance, fibroid (a type of growth in the wall of uterus), or defect in the blood clotting mechanism in young age called coagulation disorder[4]. It may also be due to vaginal infections. It is very common in adolescent girls because of slight thyroid hormonal imbalances in their age.

Excessive blood loss from body may lead to fall in the level of hemoglobin to less than 11 gm%. This condition is called anemia. More than half of the adolescent girls suffer from this condition in India. To prevent the adolescent girls should take at least one tablet of Iron and Folic acid daily on regular basis. In case of moderate anemia (hemoglobin 8-10 gm%) they should take two tablets daily for at least three months. Severe anemia (Hemoglobin <8 gm%) requires treatment in hospital. Due importance should also be give to the natural method of dealing with the problem,i.e., DIETARY MEASURES. (see chapter on anemia).

Many times adolescent girls suffer from worm infestation which makes anemia worse. Treating worm infestation can help in preventing aggravation of anemia.

Hypomenorrhea: Sometimes the flow is scanty and can be as less as a spot. But, if it is regular and is not associated with pain, there is nothing much to worry. Proper nutrition and regular physical exercise can improve the condition.

Amenorrhea is the absence or abnormal stoppage of menstruation. Girls who have attained the age of 16 years and still not started getting their periods are said to have primary amenorrhoea. It can be due to a hormonal imbalance or a developmental problem. For this they should consult a doctor. When a woman who was having normal periods suddenly stops menstruating for more than 6 months it is called secondary amenorrhea. Most common cause of secondary amenorrhea remains pregnancy.

Intermenstrual bleeding: Sometime bleeding occurs in between the due dates. It can be due to benign conditions like fibroid - a type of abnormal tumor like structure in the uterus or pelvic inflammatory diseases e.g. tubercular infection of internal reproductive organs in young age group. This is quite common condition in India. In this the cycles are regular but in between the cycles spotting occurs. But females with sexual exposure prior to such symptoms need to ensure whether they are pregnant and whether the pregnancy is outside the uterine cavity or whether incomplete abortion has occurred.

The painful, heavy, unpredictable bleeding following a period of amenorrhea is suggestive of anovulatory (eggless) cycles. This is normal in the first two years of menarche. But if it occurs along with excessive weight gain, hair growth on the face (called hirsutism) it indicates some disease. Scientific studies suggest that anovulatory cycles in women with infertility tend to occur more during those months in the year when temperature is increased [5]. If it continues the woman/girl should contact a doctor so that proper diagnosis may be made and the hormonal levels in the blood may be assessed if required. Various hormonal treatments are available which should to be started under the proper medical supervision.

Premenstrual Syndrome: Approximately 7 to 10 days before the menstrual period begins, some girls experience headaches, disturbances in mood, constipation, craving for food, weight gain, and breast tenderness. These complaints are collectively called as premenstrual syndrome (PMS). Indian studies indicate that pre-menstrual complaints are generally mild and bearable in Indian women[6]. It is common among women working in industrial setup. In menstruating women, blood calcium levels can begin to fall off about 10 days prior to the start of the menstrual period. Calcium supplements or calcium containing food and herbs are important ways to prevent PMS. Some foods and herbs that have a good amount of easily assimilated calcium are cheese, curd, butter milk, eggs and fish. The cheapest sources are green leafy vegetables (e.g spinach, amaranth). *Sita phal* and Ragi are particularly rich in calcium. Few studies have found that regular exercise can ease some amount of pain and stress that lead to PMS.

What should a girl/ woman do to have a healthy menstruation?

Even though most of the menstrual problems are self limiting, some of them may cause considerable discomfort. If following measures do not help they should consult a doctor :-

1. Good dietary habits —less intake of fatty food, daily consumption of at least 100 gm of green leafy vegetables, and adequate intake of water.
2. Yoga and meditation have proven to be beneficial in maintaining the hormonal balance and reducing stress level in human body which remain trigger factor for PMS etc.
3. Physical exercise in form of walking and aerobics help in reducing pain and lethargy related to menstruation.
4. If anyone in the family is suffering from TB he/ she should receive the full course of anti- tubercular drugs.
5. Menstrual Hygiene: i) Washing of genitalia after urination, defecation and sexual intercourse is not only a good habit but also is mandatory. It prevents many infections and diseases.
   ii) Avoidance of over soakage of pads by changing pads frequently: It is useful to prevent allergic skin reactions and infections.
   iii) Always use sanitary napkins or a new cloth in place of unclean old cloths. If you are using same cloth again and again wash it thoroughly with soap and dry it in intense sunlight.
6. Personal hygiene: Simple measures like taking bath daily, regular trimming of nails also help in preventing infections.(also see chapter on menarche)

References

1. Padubidri VG, Daftary SN, Shaw's Textbook of Gynaecology. 13th ed. New Delhi: Elsevier; 2004. p. 46.
2. Patel V, Tanksale V, Sahasrabhojanee M, Gupte S, Nevrekar P. The burden and determinants of dysmenorrhoea: a population-based

survey of 2262 women in Goa, India. BJOG. 2006 Apr;113(4): 453-63.

3. Sharma M, Gupta S. Menstrual pattern and abnormalities in the high school girls of Dharan: a cross sectional study in two boarding schools. Nepal Med Coll J. 2003 Jun;5(1): 34-6.
4. Trasi SA, Pathare AV, Shetty SD, Ghosh K, Salvi V, Mohanty D The spectrum of bleeding disorders in women with menorrhagia: a report from Western India. Ann Hematol. 2005 May;84(5): 339-42.
5. Rameshkumar K, Thomas JA, Mohammed A. Atmospheric temperature & anovulation in south Indian women with primary infertility. Indian J Med Res. 1992 Feb;96: 27-8.
6. Chaturvedi SK; Chandra PS; Gururaj G; Beena MB; Pandian RD; Prabha S Chandra Prevalence of premenstrual symptoms and syndromes: preliminary observations. NIMHANS J. 1994 Jan; 12(1): 9-14.
7. http://www.seasonsindia.com/healthfitness/premenstrual_sea.htm
8. Singh AJ. Place of Menstruation in the Reproductive Lives of Women of Rural North India. Indian Journal of Community Medicine 2006; 31:10-14.

28

Mental Health of Women

Karobi Das

Women's health is linked to their status in society. It benefits from equality, and suffers from discrimination. Today, the status and wellbeing of countless millions of women worldwide remain tragically low[1]. Databases generated by many sources include appalling statistics on women's health in general and mental health in particular. Unipolar depression among women has been named to be the second most important cause of disease burden by the year 2020 [2].

Reports of violence against women are on the increase. It scars the psyche almost permanently. Childhood sexual abuse, female infanticide in some societies, battering of female children, the psychological trauma inflicted by dowry demands on newly married women, the resulting homelessness are all sordid tales of the world's apathy, neglect and indifference. The relative lack of education and authority make them extremely vulnerable to all kinds of abuse, all of which result in increasing emotional morbidity[3].

Burden of disease and disability adjusted life years which have now been extensively studied, show the importance of mental health of women in terms of role performance, productivity and health economics. In women, neuropsychiatric conditions were the second leading cause of disease burden world wide, following infections and parasitic diseases. In women between the ages of 15 to 44 years of age, unipolar depression was the leading cause of disease burden followed by schizophrenia, bipolar disorder and obsessive-compulsive disorders.[3] The bulk of the disease burden will therefore remain in the prime child-bearing, child-rearing, parenting and working years.

From the perspective of women and mental health, the key epidemiological finding is the much replicated association of female gender and common mental disorders such as depression and anxiety. Both community based studies and studies of treatment seekers indicate that women are on average, two to three times, at greater risk to be affected by these disorders[4,5]. Findings suggest that reasons for this vulnerability is the association between stressful life events and depression [6,7]. Women are far more likely to be victims of violence in their homes. The multiple roles of child-bearing, child-rearing, caring for sick relatives, running the home, and job may lead to considerable stress.The reproductive roles of women, such as their expected roles of bearing children, the consequences of infertility and the failure to produce a male child have also been linked to wife-battering and female suicide[8,9].

The Schizophrenia Research Foundation at Chennai, India carried out an ethnographic, qualitative study of 75 mentally ill women who were separated or divorced. It was found that in 67 of these separated women lived in their parental homes with the onus of care being borne by the aging parents[10]. This study brings into focus some issues, which confront women in many developing countries.

- Lack of awareness of the illness and its disabilities resulting in the widespread belief that marriage is a remedy for all ills. This resulted in the marriages of mentally ill women and the suppression of this fact from their husbands and in – laws.
- An absence of legal protection including maintenance for such women.
- Burden of care of these women goes back to the parents, who are aging and may be sick.

- Lack of any state managed programme which would offer these women some physical, sexual and financial security.

Studies of suicide and deliberate self-harm have revealed a common trend of more female attempters and more male completers of suicide. A large number of studies have replicated them with similar findings. Studies have also shown that women married young seem to be at a higher risk for attempted suicide and self harm[11].

Reproductive health is a fundamental aspect of women's health and tends to envelop mental health issues too. Psychological issues related to childbirth, violence, rape, adverse maternal outcomes such as stillbirths and abortions, reproductive tract surgeries, sterilization, premarital pregnancies in adolescents, HIV/AIDS, menopause and infertility are all areas which cause mental health problems in women.

- In women attending gynecological clinics rates of depression reported are unusually high. A strong relationship exists between vaginal discharge, weakness, psychosomatic symptoms and psychosocial stress.
- Psychiatric admissions also show an increase during the first three months post partum. Although the blues do not require intervention, it is important to note that this syndrome appears to be a risk factor for later depression. Research indicates a wide range of prevalence of post natal depression from 3-36% of mothers after childbirth[12-15].

The sexual health of adolescents is now a major issue in reproductive health research and programmes because of the obvious potential of HIV/AIDS prevention by empowering young people to take decisions regarding their sexual health. There are other mental health problems like stress arising from conflict within families, pressures in the educational system and increasing unemployment.

Menopause is another time in the reproductive cycle that is marked by hormonal change and depression. Research suggests that there is an increase in new onset of depressive illness in women aged 45 to 50 years. The evidence supports this linkage that women with a prior history of depression are at increased risk for depression at menopause.

Gynecological surgery poses a unique stress for women because of the identification of the reproductive organs both with sexuality and with the wider concept of feminine identity[18]. This stress is particularly more so with hysterectomy. It has been associated with adverse psychological sequelae.

Women's mental health is increasingly recognized as a major public health concern with impact on the well – being of individuals, families and society.

The last two decades have witnessed a growth of self – help movements in women's groups, and some local groups have been outstanding in their efforts. Examples of this are the anti-alcohol movement by women in the state of Andhra Pradesh[3] and the activities of local men and women in Chennai during theTsunami. There is an urgent need to strongly reinforce such movements, since they are all measures which will strengthen self esteem, enhance problem solving skills and reinforce autonomy and assertiveness.

Steps to attain sound mental health

A few techniques have been enumerated below which the author has found extremely useful in helping men and women with mental health problems.

- Make a checklist of common symptoms of stress. Use it as a screening tool. It enables one to check how 'high' or 'low' one is on stress level.
- Give at least twenty minutes to YOUR SELF. You brush your teeth daily – to avoid tooth decay. Give time for self even if you haven't finished the chores for the day. Do simple physical exercises on a regular basis. Body stretching, leg and limb exercises, forward and backward bending, spinal abdominal exercises remove muscle tension, aches and pains and make the body more flexible.

Breathing exercises – help in circulation of blood and improves concentration.

- FOOD, SLEEP and WORK habits must be modulated.
- Living in the moment. Freedom from stress involves making peace with IMPERFECTION. Able to accept things as they are.
- Serving others is an effective strategy. 'The less important I feel, the less stress I harbour. Takes attention off my little world'.

- Meet the needs of socialization by being with friends who are supportive and involvement in community activities.
- Working on one's hobbies – you are so involved that you forget your problems and pain. For example, gardening – pulling out weeds – elimination of negative thoughts.
- Redirecting one's thinking
  - No news is good news
  - Out of this experience only good will come out.
  - Changing attitude
  - Under react and stay calm
- Analyse your feelings

"Person who gives me any problem that's me, I create my own feelings. I make myself more uncomfortable".

  - Do not distance yourself from them
  - Take control
  - Talk rationally to self.
  - Get organized

Develop a realistic schedule of daily activities. Time for work, sleep, relationships, recreation, home, family, daily dose of conversation and sharing of deep feelings.

- Crying is not bad.
  It is a natural response to frustrations. You feel better after crying. Helps to get rid of chemicals which if accumulated can harm us.
- Laughter is the best medicine. When you laugh the whole body benefits.
  - Lungs gets exercised
  - Heart gets extra tuning
  - Blood pressure gets lowered
  - Breathing becomes easier
  - Sound sleep is induced
- Everybody needs someone – to talk to, to hold, to cuddle, to be with and to share emotions. Caring and sharing improves emotional health.
- Deal with anger positively. It is an emotional response. Anger is dangerous when allowed to build up inside. Don't hide it nor should you go and hit someone. Get away from anger through sportsand exercise.

- Develop a faith factor.
    - Spirituality.
    - It is not religious dogma, rather a supreme way of life.
    - Ethical awareness, control over sense organs, restraint and renunciation, humility, love, gentleness, selflessness, fearlessness, forgiveness, tranquility, relaxation and equanimity of mind.
    - It does not imply that we renounce all worldly things.
    - It implies a life of peace, faith in self and others, hope, compassion freedom from anxiety and insecurity.
    - Enhances our ability to cope with stress and illness.

References

1. The World Health Report. World Health Organization, 1998, Geneva.
2. United Nations Development Programme, Human Development Report. 1977, New York, Oxford University Press.
3. Thara. R., Patel V., Women's Mental Health: A Public Health Concern, Regional Health Forum, 5(1), 2000, 24-33.
4. Patel V., Araya R., Lima, M.S., Ludermir A., Todd C., Women, Poverty and common mental disorders in four restructuring societies. Social Science and Medicine, 1999, 49; 1461-71.
5. Mumford DB, Saeed K., Ahmad I., Latif S., Mubbashar M., Stress and psychiatric disorder in rural Punjab. A community survey. British J of Psychiatry, 1997, 170 : 473-78.
6. Hussain N, Creed F., Tomenson B., Depression and Social Stress in Pakistan. Psychological Medicine 2000, 30 : 395-402.
7. Listening to women talk about their Health : Issues and Evidence from India, 1994. New Delhi, Ford Foundation.
8. Davar B., The Mental Health of Indian Women : A Feminist Agenda, 1999, New Delhi, Sage (India).
9. Dennerstein L., Astbury J., Morse C., Psychosocial and Mental Health Aspects of Women's Health WHO/FHE/MNH/93.1, 1993 World Health Organization.
10. SCARF publication. A study of Mentally disabled women, 1998.
11. Biswas S., Roy S., Debnath C., Sengupta S.B., A Study of attempted suicide in adolescents in West Bengal, Indian Journal of Psychiatry, 1997, 39 : 54-55.

12. Kennerly, H., and Gath D., Maternity blues : Assocaition with Obstetric, psychological and psychiatric factors, British J of Psychiatry, 1989, 155: 367-373.
13. O' Hara, M.W. Post partum mental disorders. In N. Droegemeuller & J. Sciarra (eds.), Gynaecology an Obstetric , 1991, Vol. 6., 1-13, Philadelphia, Lippincott.
14. Gautam S., Nijhawan M., Gehlot P., Post partum psychiatric syndromes : an analysis of 100 cases. Indian Journal of Psychiatry, 1982, 24 : 383-6.
15. Kit, L.K., Janet G., Jegasothy R., Incidence of Post natal depression in Malaysian women Journal of Obstetric & Gynaecological Research, 1997, 23: 85-89.
16. Das K., and Kohli A., Psychology of women, 2007, Women and Society, New Delhi., Global vision Publishing Hsouse.

29

Mental Health Problems of Women: Nonpharmacological Interventions

S K Mattoo and Shubh Mohan Singh

Introduction

The World Health Organization (WHO) defines health as a state of complete physical, mental and social well being and not merely absence of disease or infirmity (1). Every woman, man, and child is said to have the human right to the highest attainable standard of physical and mental health, without discrimination of any kind (2). However, inequities in the distribution of health resources remain (3) and gender is a particularly potent determinant of such inequity (4).

The importance of mental health enshrined in the WHO definition of health (1), is underlined by the enormous burden caused by the mental disorders (5). This burden includes the cost of medical treatment in view of the prolonged and/or recurrent nature of most of the common psychiatric disorders. The globalization of the pharmaceutical industry has begun to increase the cost in developing countries, often making it unaffordable for the poorer sections of the society. In addition, the inequities for mental health resource allocation are glaring (6) and are compounded by the relative lack of good quality data regarding low-cost and effective interventions for mental disorders in developing countries (7). Therefore, research needs to focus on alternate-nonmedical, traditional, and informal interventions that are low-cost, and easy to avail and administer (7).

Generally, all over the world women are central to wage earning, agriculture and other production activities and home management, roles which are sadly neglected and often glossed over (8). A woman is also at a disadvantage when accessing mental health services vis-à-vis men (9). High-cost interventions are likely to be poorly accessed by a majority of women in the country. This chapter attempts to provide an outline of low-cost, particularly non-pharmacological interventions for mental disorders across the life cycle of women particularly in developing countries like India.

An Overview of Epidemiology of Major Mental Disorders in Women (Fig. 1)

Significant differences exist between males and females with relation to mental disorders. In general, women are 5-7 years older at age of onset of symptoms of schizophrenia than men (10). There is also a significant increase in the incidence of first episode psychosis in women aged 45-49 years (11). While women may suffer less from substance abuse and personality disorders, they have about 1.5 times higher lifetime prevalence of mood disorders (24% vs 15%) and anxiety disorders (30% vs 19%). The ratio of depressed women to men is 2:1 across all cultures and the incidence increases with the child-bearing age and is intimately associated with stressful life events and lack of autonomy (12-14).

Schizophrenias and Other Psychoses in Women

Schizophrenia is a chronic and disabling mental disorder. Although the mainstay of treatment is with antipsychotic agents, increasingly pharmacotherapy is being complemented with psychosocial approaches, to good results (15). The foremost aim of any psychosocial intervention in schizophrenia is to impart psychoeducation to enhance care-giver's knowledge and medication compliance and this has been shown to significantly reduce relapse (16). Patient and family education, and community based interventions to ensure re-entry of patients into mainstream have also shown to improve results significantly (17, 18).

However, problems remain for women due to the structure of the society that we live in. Traditionally, help for families with schizophrenia has focused on family of origin and this may not be appropriate for women who do not live with their parents. Specific interventions are required focusing on the patient as a mother who may be bewildered by the emotional numbing experience of the negative symptoms of schizophrenia or the husband who as the primary caregiver may be put in an unfamiliar role (17). It has also been seen that psychoeducation imparted to family members has a gender specific absorption with females tending to gain more than males. The obvious lesson is that psychoeducation is more likely to be helpful when imparted to a significant female in the current household of the woman (18).

Case Study - 1

Six months into her marriage Beena started showing sexually disinhibited behavior. She claimed to be the incarnation of the most-beautiful-ever-woman Rani Roopmati on the basis of voices that only she (none else) could hear. When contradicted she turned abusive and violent and started accusing everyone of being against her and out to kill her. She ate only food cooked by her self. She laughed and wept loudly for no reason, and neglected her work and personal care. A local qualified doctor diagnosed her to be suffering from schizophrenia and treated her with medication. She recovered in a few months. Assuming she had been cured she stopped her medication, despite the advice of the doctor and her family against it. Within a few weeks her abnormal behavior relapsed. This relapse and further advice of the doctor to continue treatment for many years made her family to ensure she continued her medication, resulted in many more years of freedom from this psychotic illness. ***Support of her family to ensure her continued medication for many years was the key to her sustained recovery.***

Depression and Anxiety

Depression tends to be a disabling and recurring condition characterized by clinically significant sadness of mood, anhedonia, lethargy, and a host of other symptoms, and causes an enormous disease burden among the women and their families. Depression and anxiety often co-occur in women and are termed as common mental disorders (19). The differences in the epidemiology of depression between men and women and significant and multifactorial (20). These disorders in women are intimately associated with adverse childhood experiences, role limitation associated with lack of choice and autonomy, competing social roles, adverse life events, and poor social support (20). Such situations are very common in low to middle income male-centric countries such as India. Some of these predisposing factors can be surmounted by empowerment of women (21).

Randomized controlled trials for non-pharmacological measures for women with depression living in developing countries are scarce. At the community level there is some support for the effectiveness: of group interpersonal psychotherapy in Uganda (22), individual problem-solving combined with medication (Fluoxetine) in India (23), multi-component stepped care including psychoeducation in Chile (24), and individual counseling sessions by minimally trained counselors in Pakistan (25). These attempts may be considered extensions of traditional social healing mechanisms. However, in all fairness it must be stressed that it is often more difficult to find trained personnel to conduct psychotherapy in the community than it is to train the basic health worker in the use of psychotropic medication.

As per the ICD-10, depression is clinically subtyped into mild, moderate and severe depression and a milder, chronic state of depression also known as dysthymia (26). For patients with dysthymia, mild depression and (in selected patients with) moderate depression non-pharmacological methods of intervention can be tried with benefit (27). In women, if assessment has indicated the presence of abuse, unresolved issues in relation to stressful life events, lack of opportunities and poor social support, then psychotherapeutic measures in particular and non-pharmacological measures in general prove useful (27). Non-pharmacological interventions may be useful in women who are pregnant, lactating or wishing to become pregnant. In countries with better infrastructure, support groups for women dealing with abuse for instance are invaluable (28).

Some **initial interventions** for depressive and anxiety disorders include education focused at clarifying the patient's uncertainty and misconceptions. Handouts and information pamphlets, if available, are useful. Information about depression should include the following:

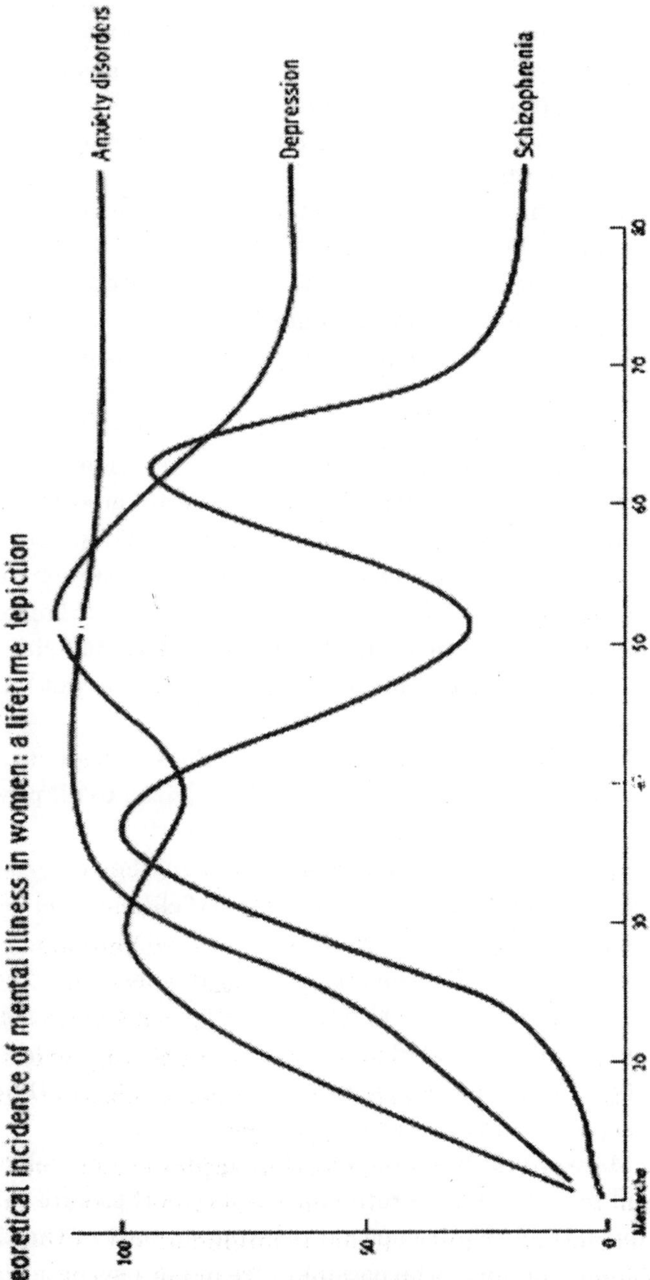
Theoretical incidence of mental illness in women: a lifetime depiction
Anxiety disorders
Depression
Schizophrenia
Incidence of mental illness (hypothetical units)
100
50
0
Menarche
20
30
50
60
70
80
Age (years)

1. Major depression is not a weakness of character but an illness like any other. This is especially important in women who may think of their own inadequacies in the wake of depression, and this may lead to further loss of self-esteem and increase in symptoms of depression.
2. Recovery is the rule rather than exception, and effective treatments exist.
3. The goal of treatment is to feel 100% better and be better equipped for the future.

Lifestyle changes are known to be effective in countering depression. These changes include:

1. *Stress management* by various behavioral and cognitive methods.
2. *Reducing drug and alcohol abuse* as these are known to be associated with increased rates of depression (29), and also to improve sleep patterns which may be an important adjunct in the non-pharmacological management of depression (30).
3. *A balanced diet* which includes complex carbohydrates and vitamins as there is some evidence that carbohydrate rich food may improve mood (31). However, this should not be taken to the extreme as some patients may put on too much weight.
4. *Regular physical exercise* like aerobics or yoga may be useful in mood elevation and should be advised to all physically fit women (32).
5. *Problem solving* treatment has been shown to be effective and feasible in both community and clinic-based populations and is especially relevant in women where life stresses play an important association with depression (33). Patient satisfaction is high and there is a low drop-out rate with this modality of treatment (33) involving problem goals, brainstorming to generate solutions, selecting the preferred solution and evaluating progress.

More **specialized psychotherapies** exist as well which may be used in mild to moderate depression. As these are manualized therapies, they require special training on part of the therapists, which may not always be possible. The major psychotherapies that are widely accepted as being effective in depressive disorders are cognitive behavior therapy (CBT) and interpersonal therapy (IPT). CBT is based on the premise that a patient's negative thoughts lead to a negative appraisal of themselves, the future and the world (34). CBT aims to change negative thoughts from distorting the patient's cognitions and resultant behaviors. CBT is delivered in 16-20 sessions over 12-16 weeks (27) and meta-analyses seem to suggest that CBT may be as or more efficacious than antidepressants (35).

IPT is a focused time-limited treatment of approximately 16 sessions which emphasize current interpersonal relationships. The therapy aims to rectify what are postulated as the reasons for depression, namely role confusion, social isolation, grief and role transition. (36). In this therapy, the therapist and the patient work together to identify interpersonal difficulties that are causing, exacerbating or maintaining depression. IPT has been considered effective in treatment of depression (36).

If after 4-8 weeks of treatment, moderate improvement has not been attained then it is important to review the case thoroughly and to plan alternative treatment modalities. Exacerbation of symptoms and presence of psychotic symptoms are indicators for institution of somatic therapies (27).

As a young bride Uma was pained to see her husband drink alcohol everyday. Her parents-in-law, the only other members of the household, were very supportive of her. Despite this her distress continued while in 6 years she become a mother of three children. After the birth of the third child she decided to stop talking to him about his drinking. However, she worried a lot and often became sad and wept; any bad news made her weep easily. The company of her children and neighbors and good news would cheer her up only briefly. Otherwise she remained anxious and startled easily. She developed frequent headaches. A local nurse advised her to see a doctor, but she did not do so and continued with her suffering. Then both her parents-in-law died in quick succession and she was left without their emotional support. Against her expectations, her husband increased his drinking. She was devastated. For many months she worried all the time, became sad, cried frequently, stopped talking to others, lost her sleep and appetite, lost weight, became hopeless. When she attempted suicide, the local doctor diagnosed her to be suffering from depression. He prescribed her antidepressants and sleeping pills, which gave her quick relief; but when she discontinued, she relapsed as quickly. At this juncture the doctor and the nurse together put her on medication again, and persuaded and referred her husband for specialist medical treatment for his alcohol problem. While her husband stopped his drinking, their problems were reviewed in detail. She was urged to continue her medication on a long-term basis, which gave her partial relief from her depression. She was advised to supervise her husband's medication, increase her participation in local religious and social activities, and talk her problems out with the local nurse/friends. Her husband and the eldest daughter agreed to take over some of her household responsibilities, while she went out to the community. With these changes in her life, she felt a lot better even though she still felt sad and anxious from time to time, more so if there was any bad news or event.

CASE VIGNET - DOUBLE DEPRESSION IN A POOR/ ALCOHOLIC FARMER'S WIFE; COPING THROUGH HELP FROM ANGANWARI WORKER/DOCTOR/SPECIALIST CARE FOR BOTH – CHANGE OF LIFE STYLE.

Pre-Menstrual Dysphoric Disorder (PMDD)

PMDD is a symptom cluster that is absent in the follicular phase of the menstrual cycle and is characterized by affective and physical symptoms in the week before the menstrual cycle. These symptoms include anxiety, irritability, depressed mood and affective lability (26). A small study on Indian women reported prevalence of 6.4% (37). The negative impact of these symptoms has been documented and the burden established (38). PMDD has been shown to be associated with hormonal factors, young age, cultural determinants of expression and severity, stressful life events and sexual abuse (39).

The non-pharmacological interventions that have been shown useful in PMDD are outlined below.

1.For women with mild symptoms, *education about the condition, supportive counseling, and general measures such as regular exercise and a balanced diet* are useful. For all patients presenting with PMDD, these measures should be advised while daily ratings necessary for the diagnosis of PMDD are done (40).

Patients should be encouraged to reduce or eliminate intake of salty food, sugar, coffee, red meat and alcohol. Increased intake of green leafy vegetables, legumes and water is recommended. Eating smaller, more frequent meals that are high in carbohydrates may be useful for symptoms of depression and anxiety (41). Aerobic exercise for 20-30 minutes and weight reduction to within 20% of ideal has also been shown to be effective (41). It is also useful to have a regular timetable and to adhere to regular bed times and waking times (41). Stressful activities that are known to exacerbate symptoms of PMDD should be avoided if possible (41).

2. *Dietary supplements* have little scientific evidence but there are anecdotal and lay-press reports that supplementation with calcium (1200mg/day) reduces symptoms of depression (42). There is also some evidence regarding efficacy of vitamin B6 (43) and vitamin E (44).

3. Psychotherapy and *group support* is also considered useful but has a scanty evidence base. Only one randomized controlled trial has examined the efficacy of CBT versus pharmacotherapy in the treatment of PMDD (45). The results indicate that CBT is as effective as medication (20mg/day of Fluoxetine), helps in improving partner relationships, daily functioning and mood, and the improvement is more sustained (45). (please also see the chapter on menstruation/adolescent health)

Infertility, Induced Abortion and Pregnancy Loss

Lack of conception after one year of unprotected sex indicates infertility (46) which tends to psychologically affect women more with decreased self-esteem and femininity. Being prolonged, costly and complicated, treatment of infertility complicates the matters. Though infertility is not known to be directly associated with major depression (47), it does cause a negative emotional state and may exacerbate a preexisting psychiatric disorder. For mild and moderate depressive and anxiety states, psychotherapeutic maneuvers as described earlier may be useful. Group psychotherapy is reported to be useful as infertility is often associated with a sense of isolation from child-bearing and rearing peers (48). A therapist may successfully persuade the partners to enter therapy and/or explore parenting options like adoption.

Similarly, induced abortion for whatever reason, may lead to guilt, self-blame or even Major depression; a history of depression during pregnancy is the strongest predictor for depression (49). A pre-abortion counseling is a must, especially with a background of contraceptive failure, rape, incest, or fetal congenital anomaly. All women with pregnancy loss, especially with a past history of infertility, should be thoroughly assessed for feelings of guilt and self-reproach (50). Based on symptom severity, such states must be managed with psychotherapy, pharmacotherapy or both.

Depression in Pregnancy

Pregnancy has traditionally been considered a time of protection against mental disorders; however this point of view is now changing. Post-partum blues for instance is very common and may affect as many as 85% of new mothers (51). Of the major mental disorders, depression associated with pregnancy is amenable to non-pharmacologic measures of intervention. Depression has a prevalence of approximately 10% in pregnant women and approximately 13-28% in postpartum women (52, 53). Depression is particularly significant in women with past history of depression, particularly in setting of antidepressant discontinuation.

The evidence base for psychotherapy in antenatal depression is scarce (54). IPT is the preferred mode of psychotherapy in such cases given the obvious relevance of interpersonal relationships and role transitions in pregnancy (55). IPT has been shown to be efficacious in antenatal depression (55). The recent Cochrane review on this topic also confirmed the paucity of data in this area and no recommendation was made in this meta-analysis (56). An interesting study from Pakistan showed the benefit of a community level, CBT-based intervention for women with perinatal depression (57). There is a more robust evidence base for the role of psychotherapy in postpartum depression (58). As per the guidelines, psychotherapy with CBT and IPT should be the first line treatment in all cases with mild to moderate postpartum depression (58). Evidence exists for group therapy in addition to individual psychotherapy as well (59).

In general, all pregnant women should be educated about the possibilities of feelings of inadequacy, low self esteem and efficacy, and should be cautioned not to feel guilty about them but to seek professional help. Psychotherapy should be offered to patients with mild to moderate depression and all those with more severe symptoms and with psychotic symptoms should be treated with somatic therapies.

Menopausal Mood Disturbances

Menopause is a time of transition that is frequently uncomfortable and distressing due to symptoms such as hot flushes, sleep disturbances, cognitive symptoms and mood disturbances (60). Evidence base for non-pharmacological methods of intervention in patients with distressing symptoms of menopause is scarce (61). However, there is evidence to suggest that some behavioral measures may be useful. These include aerobic exercise, health education regarding menopause, and paced respiration (61).

Rape, Violence and Assault

Sexual assault on women is considered to be commoner than that reported. The psychological sequelae of rape may range from initial symptoms of shock, followed by autonomic hyper-arousal to delayed sequelae of sexual aversion, depression, post traumatic stress disorder etc. (62). Assessment should focus on presenting symptoms, preassault level of functioning, and the available support system. If needed, provisions should be made for short-term safety. Pre-existing psychiatric disorders should be treated aggressively to prevent further decompensation. One should be non-judgmental and openly supportive at all times to provide for a 'psychological debriefing'. Medication may be required to counter symptoms of anxiety, depression and dissociation. Initial symptoms that disappear with time, may recur at future times of (similar) stress. Hence, continued support must be assured and provided.

Tara was returning alone from her evening tuition when a heavy downpour stopped her for two hours. When she restated it was already dark and isolated. Soon she realized a middle-aged man was walking behind her, trying to get close. When she tried to run he chased her, caught her and tried to persuade her for sex with him. When he resisted he became more insistent, aggressive and violent, and tried to rape her. She fought back, raised an alarm and was lucky that some nearby people rescued her and overpowered the fleeing culprit. The police was called in, she was escorted back home, and a case was registered against the criminal. Even though saved from the rape Tara found her predicament unbearable. She had become the centre of unwanted attention from the neighbors, class-/school-mates, people in general and the media. Everybody wanted to talk to her about the finer details of the incident which she found shameful. She started remaining aloof, anxious and sad; had terrifying dreams at night; would startle very easily during the day; lost appetite, sleep, and interest in studies and all that was pleasurable for her earlier -radio, TV, cinema, singing, and chatting with her family and friends. Worse was to come when she was interrogated by the police and asked questions that she found extremely embarrassing; including hints that somehow she was responsible for the incident / inviting the attack on her. She started considering herself to be guilty, had frequent weeping spells and suicidal thoughts so as to get out of the situation once for all. A social worker attached with the police for cases like hers was very understanding. She spent quite some time with Tara enquiring after how she felt about her ordeal. She persuaded Tara to seek a consultation with a trained counselor. The counselor had a few sessions with Tara and persuaded her to stop feeling guilty about the incident and resolve to face the situation boldly. Tara felt better but her sadness and anxiety would not go away. The counselor referred her to a psychiatrist who prescribed some medications and advised her to continue to see the counselor who taught her some methods of relaxation including some yoga. Over many months of medication and counseling Tara was able to overcome the trauma, and feel psychologically stable enough to start enjoying her life as previously. Gradually her medication was stopped while for many years she continued with the counseling in which the counselor helped her to understand her reactions to this event in the context of her lifetime experiences, and how to change those reactions appropriately. However, stressful events and situations continued to very easily upset her. On the whole, a combination of medication and long-term psychotherapy had greatly helped her stabilize and put her life back on a smoother forward journey.

Women-specific Cancers

Women specific cancers involve the breast and gynecological cancers. These are particularly stressful as they impinge on the sense of self and identity as a woman, in addition to the stress of treatment or a sense of lack of control. A psychiatric consultation may be required for such cases. Guided imagery and progressive relaxation techniques are often useful, with or without adjunctive benzodiazepine treatment. Sleep hygiene review is often useful for problematic nighttime sleep. Psychotherapy and group support in such cases where surgery has been extensive improve survival rates (63).

Shabira had a breast lump which was diagnosed as a cancer. She was devastated by the diagnosis. Even after being operated and treated with anti cancer medications which caused her very distressing side effects, her doctors would not say that she had been cured of the illness. She could not make her doctors to say that her cancer would not kill her in ten, or even five years. She felt very depressed and suicidal till she met Sudha, whose life circumstances were almost similar except that she was still leading a cheerful life. Shabira was intrigued. She asked Sudha and was surprised to find the reason for this. Sudha was running a group which helped the cancer survivors and their families. All her 'free' time was spent in helping others while Shabira was constantly wallowing in her personal grief. Urged by Sudha, Shabira became a part of her group. A few months later, one day she suddenly realized that unlike her previous sad self she was laughing and enjoying her life unmindful of the fact that it was going to be no more than just a few years. She reminded herself that her life had changed for the better because she had asked Sudha a question and then agreed to accept her advice to follow in her footsteps.

What Works in Non-Pharmacological Interventions in Women

From the foregoing discussion, it is clear that there is a definite role of non-pharmacological interventions in common mental disorders of women. However, the mechanism of what works in such interventions is unclear. At the very least, certain common points can be discerned which may then be used in individual case management by workers in the field who may not have access to training in manualized, formal psychotherapy. These common points are as follows:

1.*Rapport*: Rapport has been defined as an "emotional resonance" with the patient. Leaving aside the merits and demerits of this definition, it does indicate a need to be able to deal with the patient on the level of the patient. In other words, it is important that the patient be able to talk with the therapist knowing that she can communicate her concerns and issues effectively and to someone who would understand in a non-patronizing and empathic manner. This should also include the ability to empathize and understand emotion expressed by the patient. An ideal candidate for such a role may be someone from the community that the patient originates from; such a person would necessarily share the concerns of the patient and be able to empathize with personal or social issues that may be perceived as stressors by the patient.

2.*Explaining the Illness*: Each school of psychology would explain a certain aspect of human psyche from its own viewpoint. A social to common-sense approach to understanding of a common mental disorder such as depression or anxiety is expected to be as effective a case formulation as any other. It is essential to develop a case-formulation because this is the pivot around which further psychotherapeutic work would revolve. For instance, a depressed woman with significant stressors in marital relation ships may need interventions at the level of family and at a personal level may be usefully helped by general principles of increasing self-efficacy and increasing sense of achievement in her own role in the family.

3.*Motivation for Therapy*: Psychotherapy is often construed as something mysterious and it is often assumed that the therapist will be the giver of new, unique and life-changing information. In reality, most modes of psychotherapy are rooted in common-sense approach to solutions of problems which are often not followed up in a sustained or organized manner. Therefore, it would be essential to make clear at the outset to dampen very high hopes and to make clear that it is not essential that circumstances would change, the change would have to come with the way those circumstances are coped with. Often patients are disheartened by the process of such interventions, at which time it is essential to explain again the nature of the intervention and the nature of the problem and thus, enhance motivation. It is also essential to adapt techniques to the needs of the patient by which highly structured and regimentalized approaches are eschewed in confused patients in favor of more free-flowing modes of intervention.

4. *Confrontation*: When a good rapport has been developed, confrontation can be gainfully used to accelerate the process of change by means of affect arousal. Affect arousal that accompanies confrontation is often associated with more learning, which can subsequently be used for therapeutic effect. For instance, confrontation of long-held beliefs of lack of autonomy may in selected patients be useful in increasing self-confidence. Here it should be stressed that though as long as possible, the patient's belief system should be respected, it is occasionally desirable that it be challenged when it proves to be an impediment in course of therapy.

5. *Goals of Therapy*: The goals of therapy should not be too ambitious as this may lead to disappointment both in the patient and the therapist. The goal should be to take the patient to a point where she can reasonably manage situation that she earlier could not and to avoid dependency on the therapist from developing.

6. *Recognition of Failure*: It is essential that the therapist recognizes worsening in the patient and not be tardy in referring the patient to more specialist care.

Conclusions

Non-pharmacological methods of intervention in women with major mental disorders and also disorders specific to women are valuable adjuncts and at times preferred methods of interventions. It is the need of the hour to develop a more robust evidence-base for these interventions especially in developing countries.

References

1. WHO. Constitution of the World Health Organization. Geneva, World Health Organization, 1948.
2. Declaration of Alma Ata. N Z Hosp. 1978 Oct;30(9):4, 6.
3. Hall JJ, Taylor R. Health for all beyond 2000: the demise of the Alma-Ata Declaration and primary health care in developing countries. Med J Aust. 2003 Jan 6;178(1):17-20.

4. Wamala S, Agren G. Gender inequity and public health. Getting down to real issues. Eur J Public Health. 2002 Sep;12(3):163-5.
5. Prince M, Patel V, Saxena S, Maj M, Maselko J, Phillips MR, et al. No health without mental health. Lancet. 2007 Sep 8;370(9590):859-77.
6. Saxena S, Thornicroft G, Knapp M, Whiteford H. Resources for mental health: scarcity, inequity, and inefficiency. Lancet. 2007 Sep 8;370(9590):878-89.
7. Patel V, Araya R, Chatterjee S, Chisholm D, Cohen A, De Silva M, et al. Treatment and prevention of mental disorders in low-income and middle-income countries. Lancet. 2007 Sep 15;370(9591):991-1005.
8. Buckshee K. Impact of roles of women on health in India. Int J Gynaecol Obstet. 1997 Jul;58(1):35-42.
9. James S, Chisholm D, Murthy RS, Kumar KK, Sekar K, Saeed K, et al. Demand for, access to and use of community mental health care: lessons from a demonstration project in India and Pakistan. Int J Soc Psychiatry. 2002 Sep;48(3):163-76.
10. Angermeyer MC, Kuhn L. Gender differences in age at onset of schizophrenia. An overview. Eur Arch Psychiatry Neurol Sci. 1988 Sep;237(6):351-64.
11. Hafner H, Maurer K, Loffler W, an der Heiden W, Munk-Jorgensen P, Hambrecht M, et al. The ABC Schizophrenia Study: a preliminary overview of the results. Soc Psychiatry Psychiatr Epidemiol. 1998 Aug;33(8):380-6.
12. Kendler KS, Karkowski-Shuman L. Stressful life events and genetic liability to major depression: genetic control of exposure to the environment? Psychol Med. 1997 May;27(3):539-47.
13. Boyd JH, Rae DS, Thompson JW, Burns BJ, Bourdon K, Locke BZ, et al. Phobia: prevalence and risk factors. Soc Psychiatry Psychiatr Epidemiol. 1990 Nov;25(6):314-23.
14. Thornicroft G, Tansella M. Components of a modern mental health service: a pragmatic balance of community and hospital care: overview of systematic evidence. Br J Psychiatry. 2004 Oct;185:283-90.
15. Ran MS, Xiang MZ, Chan CL, Leff J, Simpson P, Huang MS, et al. Effectiveness of psychoeducational intervention for rural Chinese families experiencing schizophrenia—a randomised controlled trial. Soc Psychiatry Psychiatr Epidemiol. 2003 Feb;38(2):69-75.

16. Li Z, Arthur D. Family education for people with schizophrenia in Beijing, China: randomised controlled trial. Br J Psychiatry. 2005 Oct;187:339-45.
17. Kulkarni J. Women and schizophrenia: a review. Aust N Z J Psychiatry. 1997 Feb;31(1):46-56.
18. McWilliams S HS, Mannion N, Kinsella A, O'Callaghan E. Caregiver psychoeducation for schizophrenia: is gender important? Eur Psychiatry. 2007;22(5):323-7.
19. Olfson M, Mechanic D. Mental disorders in public, private nonprofit, and proprietary general hospitals. Am J Psychiatry. 1996 Dec;153(12):1613-9.
20. Piccinelli M, Wilkinson G. Gender differences in depression. Critical review. Br J Psychiatry. 2000 Dec;177:486-92.
21. Kermode M, Herrman H, Arole R, White J, Premkumar R, Patel V. Empowerment of women and mental health promotion: a qualitative study in rural Maharashtra, India. BMC Public Health. 2007;7:225.
22. Bolton P, Bass J, Neugebauer R, Verdeli H, Clougherty KF, Wickramaratne P, et al. Group interpersonal psychotherapy for depression in rural Uganda: a randomized controlled trial. Jama. 2003 Jun 18;289(23):3117-24.
23. Patel V, Chisholm D, Rabe-Hesketh S, Dias-Saxena F, Andrew G, Mann A. Efficacy and cost-effectiveness of drug and psychological treatments for common mental disorders in general health care in Goa, India: a randomised, controlled trial. Lancet. 2003 Jan 4;361(9351):33-9.
24. Araya R, Rojas G, Fritsch R, Gaete J, Rojas M, Simon G, et al. Treating depression in primary care in low-income women in Santiago, Chile: a randomised controlled trial. Lancet. 2003 Mar 22;361(9362):995-1000.
25. Ali BS, Rahbar MH, Naeem S, Gul A, Mubeen S, Iqbal A. The effectiveness of counseling on anxiety and depression by minimally trained counselors: a randomized controlled trial. Am J Psychother. 2003;57(3):324-36.
26. Organization WH. International Classification of Diseases, 10th Revision (ICD-10). Geneva; 1992.
27. Society IP. Clinical practice guidleines for psychiatrists in India; 2005.
28. McArthur MJ. Reality therapy with rape victims. Arch Psychiatr Nurs. 1990 Dec;4(6):360-5.

29. Palfai TP, Cheng DM, Samet JH, Kraemer KL, Roberts MS, Saitz R. Depressive symptoms and subsequent alcohol use and problems: a prospective study of medical inpatients with unhealthy alcohol use. J Stud Alcohol Drugs. 2007 Sep;68(5):673-80.
30. Phillips B, Mannino D. Correlates of sleep complaints in adults: the ARIC study. J Clin Sleep Med. 2005 Jul 15;1(3):277-83.
31. Wurtman JJ. Depression and weight gain: the serotonin connection. J Affect Disord. 1993 Oct-Nov;29(2-3):183-92.
32. Woolery A, Myers H, Sternlieb B, Zeltzer L. A yoga intervention for young adults with elevated symptoms of depression. Altern Ther Health Med. 2004 Mar-Apr;10(2):60-3.
33. Mynors-Wallis LM, Gath DH, Lloyd-Thomas AR, Tomlinson D. Randomised controlled trial comparing problem solving treatment with amitriptyline and placebo for major depression in primary care. Bmj. 1995 Feb 18;310(6977):441-5.
34. Beck A. Cognitive therapy and emotional disorders. New York: Guilford Press; 1976.
35. Gloaguen V, Cottraux J, Cucherat M, Blackburn IM. A meta-analysis of the effects of cognitive therapy in depressed patients. J Affect Disord. 1998 Apr;49(1):59-72.
36. Zogg W. [Review of several different forms of psychotherapy in treatment of depression]. Ther Umsch. 2000 Feb;57(2):62-70.
37. Banerjee N, Roy KK, Takkar D. Premenstrual dysphoric disorder—a study from India. Int J Fertil Womens Med. 2000 Sep-Oct;45(5):342-4.
38. Chawla A, Swindle R, Long S, Kennedy S, Sternfeld B. Premenstrual dysphoric disorder: is there an economic burden of illness? Med Care. 2002 Nov;40(11):1101-12.
39. Ross LE, Steiner M. A biopsychosocial approach to premenstrual dysphoric disorder. Psychiatr Clin North Am. 2003 Sep;26(3):529-46.
40. Mitwally MF, Kahn LS, Halbreich U. Pharmacotherapy of premenstrual syndromes and premenstrual dysphoric disorder: current practices. Expert Opin Pharmacother. 2002 Nov;3(11):1577-90.
41. Frackiewicz EJ, Shiovitz TM. Evaluation and management of premenstrual syndrome and premenstrual dysphoric disorder. J Am Pharm Assoc (Wash). 2001 May-Jun;41(3):437-47.

42. Thys-Jacobs S, Starkey P, Bernstein D, Tian J. Calcium carbonate and the premenstrual syndrome: effects on premenstrual and menstrual symptoms. Premenstrual Syndrome Study Group. Am J Obstet Gynecol. 1998 Aug;179(2):444-52.

43. Wyatt KM, Dimmock PW, Jones PW, Shaughn O'Brien PM. Efficacy of vitamin B-6 in the treatment of premenstrual syndrome: systematic review. Bmj. 1999 May 22;318(7195):1375-81.

44. London RS, Murphy L, Kitlowski KE, Reynolds MA. Efficacy of alpha-tocopherol in the treatment of the premenstrual syndrome. J Reprod Med. 1987 Jun;32(6):400-4.

45. Hunter MS, Ussher JM, Browne SJ, Cariss M, Jelley R, Katz M. A randomized comparison of psychological (cognitive behavior therapy), medical (fluoxetine) and combined treatment for women with premenstrual dysphoric disorder. J Psychosom Obstet Gynaecol. 2002 Sep;23(3):193-9.

46. Lapane KL, Zierler S, Lasater TM, Stein M, Barbour MM, Hume AL. Is a history of depressive symptoms associated with an increased risk of infertility in women? Psychosom Med. 1995 Nov-Dec;57(6):509-13; discussion 14-6.

47. Downey J, McKinney M. The psychiatric status of women presenting for infertility evaluation. Am J Orthopsychiatry. 1992 Apr;62(2):196-205.

48. Domar AD, Clapp D, Slawsby E, Kessel B, Orav J, Freizinger M. The impact of group psychological interventions on distress in infertile women. Health Psychol. 2000 Nov;19(6):568-75.

49. Dagg PK. The psychological sequelae of therapeutic abortion—denied and completed. Am J Psychiatry. 1991 May;148(5):578-85.

50. Neugebauer R, Kline J, Shrout P, Skodol A, O'Connor P, Geller PA, et al. Major depressive disorder in the 6 months after miscarriage. Jama. 1997 Feb 5;277(5):383-8.

51. O'Hara MW, Schlechte JA, Lewis DA, Wright EJ. Prospective study of postpartum blues. Biologic and psychosocial factors. Arch Gen Psychiatry. 1991 Sep;48(9):801-6.

52. O'Hara MW. Social support, life events, and depression during pregnancy and the puerperium. Arch Gen Psychiatry. 1986 Jun;43(6):569-73.

53. Patel V, Rodrigues M, DeSouza N. Gender, poverty, and postnatal depression: a study of mothers in Goa, India. Am J Psychiatry. 2002 Jan;159(1):43-7.

54. McGowen KR MM. Depression treatment during pregnancy. Am J Psychiatry. 2004;161(11):2137-8.
55. Spinelli MG. Interpersonal psychotherapy for depressed antepartum women: a pilot study. Am J Psychiatry. 1997 Jul;154(7):1028-30.
56. Dennis CL, Ross LE, Grigoriadis S. Psychosocial and psychological interventions for treating antenatal depression. Cochrane Database Syst Rev. 2007(3):CD006309.
57. Rahman A. Challenges and opportunities in developing a psychological intervention for perinatal depression in rural Pakistan—a multi-method study. Arch Womens Ment Health. 2007;10(5):211-9.
58. Nonacs R, Cohen LS. Postpartum mood disorders: diagnosis and treatment guidelines. J Clin Psychiatry. 1998;59 Suppl 2:34-40.
59. Gjerdingen D. The effectiveness of various postpartum depression treatments and the impact of antidepressant drugs on nursing infants. J Am Board Fam Pract. 2003 Sep-Oct;16(5):372-82.
60. Dennerstein L, Dudley EC, Hopper JL, Guthrie JR, Burger HG. A prospective population-based study of menopausal symptoms. Obstet Gynecol. 2000 Sep;96(3):351-8.
61. NIH State-of-the-Science Conference Statement on management of menopause-related symptoms. NIH Consens State Sci Statements. 2005;22(1):1-38.
62. Kozaric-Kovacic D, Folnegovic-Smalc V, Skrinjaric J, Szajnberg NM, Marusic A. Rape, torture, and traumatization of Bosnian and Croatian women: psychological sequelae. Am J Orthopsychiatry. 1995 Jul;65(3):428-33.
63. Spiegel D, Bloom JR, Kraemer HC, Gottheil E. Effect of psychosocial treatment on survival of patients with metastatic breast cancer. Lancet. 1989 Oct 14;2(8668):888-91.

30

Nature Cures

Manju Wadwalkar

Introduction

After extensive research, modern medicine has finally recognized the importance of plant-foods. Besides vitamins and minerals, cereals, vegetables, fruits, pulses, nuts, spices, tea and wine contain useful micronutrients. These micronutrients, now considered the vitamins of 21st century, are called phytochemicals. These are the gift of nature to mankind.

Phytochemicals act as antioxidants and detoxifying agents against chronic and degenerative diseases like diabetes, cancer, cataract, cardiovascular disorders and ageing. These hidden nutrients are capable of cleaning the body of dangerous free radicals.

Free radicals play an important role in causing impaired brain function, cataract, cancer, heart diseases as well as speeding up ageing. With age, the body tissues and cells degenerate through oxidation. Free radicals play havoc with our systems and are capable of inhibiting almost all the vital functions of our body. Cancer of various organs, blood diseases like malaria, sickle cell anaemia, acute respiratory distress syndrome, atherosclerosis, myocardial infarction, ocular degeneration and Parkinson's disease are some of the adverse effects of free radicals on us.

About 200 epidemiological studies show that people who eat a lot of fruits and vegetables are less prone to cancer and ageing. These plant-based foods minimize the risk of degenerative diseases.

There are about 30,000 phytochemicals, of which at least 10,000 present in our food are derived from plants. These exist as pigments, aromatic and pungent matter as well as stimulants in various plant foods.

Phytochemicals lend colour to fruits and vegetables like mangoes, papaya, carrots, spinach, grapes, apples, cabbage, tomatoes, etc. They instill aroma in cloves, cinnamon, cardamom, fennel, cumin and turmeric, and pungency in garlic, onions, mint, ginger, lemon and pepper. In tea, coffee, wine and similar beverages, these act as stimulants.

Studies conducted by the National Institute of Nutrition (NIN) have shown that turmeric, onion and garlic contain anti-ageing, anti-inflammatory, anti-bacterial, anti-viral and anti-fungal properties. The essential oils present in spices and herbs like limonene in citrus fruits and gingerol in ginger are known to have cancer protecting effects.

The traditional Chinese medicine too relies on juices of fresh fruits, soups of herbs and vegetables, and different teas having healing properties. Specific foods are used to improve appearance, to control body weight, treat hypertension and diabetes.

Herbs for Health

The World Health Organization estimated that 80 per cent of Earth's inhabitants rely on traditional medicine for their health care. Most therapies heal patients through the use of plant extracts. Today in the US alone, the annual sale of medicinal herbs and related commodities exceeds two billion dollars. Self-prescribed preparations for cold, cough, anxiety, constipation, arthritis, fever, headaches, infections, indigestion, stress, ulcers and weakness are mostly herbal.

Ginger, garlic, turmeric, liquorice, psyllium, fenugreek, aloe vera, mint and ginseng are some of the popular medicinal herbs. Some of the culinary herbs used since ages to flavor foods are coriander, cumin, garlic, ginger, turmeric, saffron, caraway (Shahjira) and thyme.

Herbs for the Heart

A diet rich in fruits, vegetables and legumes is good for the heart. A few herbs have shown to benefit heart patients significantly.

Psyllium, commonly known as isabgol, has benefited patients with high cholesterol levels. When 5 gms of psyllium was given twice a day for four months to subjects with blood cholesterol concentrations exceeding 220 mg/d1, their cholesterol concentration dropped by an average of 13 mg/d1. Subjects consuming high fat diets too were helped greatly. Extensive research in the US, UK, India and many other countries has shown garlic to be heart-protective. Regular use of garlic reduces the risk of heart attack and stroke.

Allicin in garlic works against bacteria, molds, yeast and viruses. When allicin breaks down into various compounds there is a reduction in the platelet aggregation and increase in fibrinolytic activity (fibrin causes blood clotting; thus, preventing internal bleeding). Researchers in Kuwait found that a daily intake of 3 gms of garlic decreases coronary heart disease in middle-aged men by 20 per cent. Lemon grass oil and fenugreek powder also lower the cholesterol content in blood, thus protecting the heart.

Anti-Cancer Herbs

Onions, garlic, mint, basil, thyme, turmeric, ginger, coriander, cumin, anise, fennel and parsley are some of the herbs identified by the National Cancer Institute (NCI) of the US as having anti-cancer properties. These herbs contain cancer protective phytochemicals. Scientists at the NCI have concluded from various studies that consumption of garlic, onion and other allium species inversely affects the occurrence of stomach cancer. In Northern China, where garlic is abundantly produced, the lowest incidence of stomach cancer is indicated. Chinese who fell under the category of 'highest intake' of allium species like garlic and onions showed 40 per cent lower incidence of stomach cancer than those who were in the 'lowest intake' category. In a Dutch study, gastroenteritis subjects consuming the highest amount of onions (at least half an onion a day) showed 50 per cent lower rate of stomach cancer. The American Chemical Society published studies where turmeric has shown to suppress the growth of stomach and skin tumours. The antioxidant element present in turmeric works as an anti-inflammatory agent in humans.

Herbs for the Immune System

Flavonoids present in herbs have pigments that promote human health and fight against microbes that cause diseases. These antioxidants work as anti-inflammatory and anti-tumour agents thus enhancing the immune function of the body. The commonly used herbs that provide flavonoids are green tea, garlic, thyme, onions, and licorice. Glycyrrhizin, a sweet component of licorice (mulethi) root has reported to increase the body activity against infections and allergies. A Japanese study has reported that the chalcones in licorice produce anti-viral activity against HIV. Traditional Indian medicine uses licorice root for various ailments.

Natural Home Remedies

Ayurveda very strongly recommends herbal medicine for many ailments. Dravya Guna and Charak Samhita are two ancient books amongst many full of such remedies. Following are some of the well known home remedies found in the traditional medicine for the following common ailments:

1. Abdominal pain

- Steep 1 tbsp mint (pudina) leaves to 1 teacup of water for sometime and take it 2-3 times in a day.
- Make a paste of equal quantities of dry coriander seeds, ginger and grated coconut. Add little salt. Eat with rice or plain chapatti.
- If the pain is around the navel grind 1 tbsp each of ajwain and dried ginger into a fine powder. Add a little black salt. Take 1 tsp of this mixture with1 teacup warm water frequently and avoid solid food.
- If the pain is due to retention of urine add ½ tsp camphor and 1 tbsp sandalwood paste to 1 tbsp warm mustard oil. Massage gently over the lower abdomen.

2. Acidity

- Chew a few holy basil (tulsi) leaves to get relief from burning and gas.
- Eat watermelon, banana or cucumber every hour.
- Drink coconut water 4-5 times a day.
- Drink a glass of cold milk for fast relief of heartburn and acidity.

- Grind well ½ tsp each of the dried rind of amla and harad. Add 1 teacup of water and boil the mixture well. Filter and drink along with 1 tsp honey.

3. Acne

- Mix 1tbsp of lime juice in 1 tbsp finely ground cinnamon powder and apply on affected areas frequently.
- A couple of garlic cloves, crushed and rubbed several times a day on the affected areas.
- Fine paste of turmeric applied on the affected areas.
- Make a paste of 1 tbsp each sandalwood and turmeric powder in a little water and apply.

4. Anaemia

- Soak 8 to 10 almonds and 1 tsp rice overnight. Remove the outer skin. Grind into a fine paste. Mix in some milk and a pinch of turmeric powder. Boil and drink along with sugar candy.
- Mix 1 tbsp juice of amla with a ripe mashed banana and eat twice or thrice a day.
- Dissolve ground cinnamon (1 tsp) and 2 tsp honey in 2 cups pomegranate juice. Dosage ½tea cup.
- Frequent intake of coriander tea- boil or steep 2 tsp coriander powder in a glass of water. Add sugar and milk to taste.
- 2 tsp fenugreek seeds cooked with 1 cup rice. Eaten with a little salt regularly for a fortnight.
- Eat papayas frequently.
- Boil 6tsp each of crushed saunf and red rose petals in 11/2 teacup water and strain. Take twice daily.
- Take 1 tsp each raw turmeric juice and honey mixed together every morning.
- Mix 2 tbsp each honey and the juice of carrot and drink for a few days.

5. Anxiety

- Remove seeds from fresh fruits of amla and grind the pulp into a fine paste. Tie it in a muslin cloth and squeeze out the juice. Take 2 tsp of this juice and mix it with two teaspoonfuls each honey and lime juice. Add to it 1 teacup water and drink on an empty stomach every morning. Whenever fresh fruits are not available, dried amla can be used. Soak 1 tbsp the previous night in a cup of water. The following morning, add 1/8 tsp finely ground black pepper powder and 2 tsp lime juice. Dilute it if necessary with water and drink every morning regularly on an empty stomach (the treatment should be continued for at least 120 days to achieve expected results).

6. Appetite loss

- Mix and powder equal quantities of ajwain, saunf, dried ginger, salt and caraway (Shahjira) seeds. Mix a teaspoon of this powder in cooked rice along with ghee and eat frequently.
- Clean some Bel leaves and grind into a paste. Take ½ tsp every morning for three days.
- One inch piece of dried ginger is cut into small pieces and boiled in 2 cups water. After mixing it with milk and sugar, take it frequently like tea.
- Half tsp ground pepper mixed with 1 tbsp jaggery powder to be taken.
- Rasam, either drunk or with plain, steamed rice.

  Rasam, the hot and tangy soup of southern cuisine can be used as a medicinal formulation, based on the permutation and combination of its constituent spices and condiments.

Step 1: grind the following: ½ tsp each cumin seeds, black pepper, coriander seeds, seedless tamarind pulp, curry leaves, garlic paste and ginger paste along with 1 ripe finely cut tomato and a little water. Boil well.

Step II: Fry ½ tsp mustard seeds along with a pinch of asafetida in 1 tsp ghee till it splutters. Add to the boiled mixture. Eat with plain steamed rice.

7. Arthritis

- Combine 6 tsps each ginger and caraway (Shahjira) seeds along with 3 tsp black pepper into a fine powder and preserve. Take ½ tsp with water twice daily.
- For arthritis with pain in limbs mix equal quantity of onion juice with warm mustard oil and apply on the affected parts.
- For arthritic swellings apply fresh milk of fig tree (latex) on the affected areas.
- Carrot leaves are to be included in the daily diet.

- Cut the castor leaves into thin shreds. Fry them in hot castor oil. Apply on the affected parts when bearably hot.

8. Asthma

- Pour 1 ½ cups hot water over 1 tsp ground ginger. Take 1 tsp lukewarm at bedtime.
- A mixture of juices of ginger and pomegranate mixed with honey, all in equal quantity. Take 1 tbsp frequently.
- Powder of equal quantities of dried ginger, pepper and long pepper, to be taken thrice daily (it can be mixed with honey or can be added to tea). 1 tsp dosage
- Take 3 or 4 small vasaka leaf-buds and chew together with a small piece of ginger for 40 days.
- Mix together ½ cup each of the juices of vasaka leaves, mint (pudina) leaves, ginger (after removing any sediment) and lime in a porcelain bowl. Add 1 cup ajwain and mix again. Leave out under the sun till the mixture is dried thoroughly. Powder and preserve in a glass jar. Dosage: ¼ tsp powder with 1 tsp honey, twice daily for a month.

9. Bad breath

- Make an infusion of 1 tsp each of cardamom, cinnamon and bay leaves in 1 teacup water. Drink it (also, cleanse the mouth with liquorice powder and chew some saunf frequently).
- Gargle with an infusion of the tulsi (sweet basil).
- Drink lime juice in warm water after frequent gargling. Repeat.
- Soak 2 tsp senna leaves in 1 glass of boiling water and use the infusion as a mouthwash.
- A mixture of equal quantities of fine salt and pepper powder, thoroughly massaged over the gums.

10. Baldness

- Fenugreek seeds, ground in water and applied on the head. Allow to soak at least 40 mts. before washing. Every morning for a month.
- Grind 1 tbsp root pieces of liquorice in 1 teacup milk with ¼ tsp saffron. Apply this paste on bald patches at bedtime continuously.

- Boil 1 teacup mustard oil with 4 tbsp henna leaves, gradually added. Filter and bottle. Massage on the bald patches regularly.
- Grind the remains of tobacco smoked in a hookah and add to boiling mustard oil. Cool and store. Massage on the bald patches regularly.
- Mix 2 teacups salt and 4 tbsp pepper powder in ½ teacup lime juice. Leave it under the sun for 3 days to dry out thoroughly. Once dry, powder and bottle. Dose: 1 tsp mixed in water, applied on bald patches at bed time. Wash off the next morning. (note : Avoid using any soap or shampoo).

11. Biliousness, stomach problems

- Fenugreek leaves, boiled and fried in butter and eaten twice daily.
- Fry 1 tsp dried neem flowers in 1 tsp ghee and mix with 1 teacup boiled rice and eat twice or thrice a day.
- Mix 1 tsp each fresh juice of mint and lime along with 1 tbsp honey. Take 3 times a day.
- Grind some tender tamarind leaves into a fine paste. Add a little salt and cooked rice.
- if there is vomiting also, Mix 1 tsp finely powdered curry leaf tree bark in 2 teacups cold water and take 2 or 3 times.
- Half tsp ginger juice with 1 tsp each fresh lime and mint (pudina) juice mixed with a tbsp of honey, taken frequently.

12. Black heads

- Mix 1tsp of lime juice in 1 tsp finely ground cinnamon powder and apply it on affected areas frequently.
- Express the juice from fresh leaves of drumstick and apply on the affected areas frequently.
- Mix 1 tsp each turmeric paste and juice of fresh coriander leaves and apply daily as a face pack before going to sleep. (Also avoid fatty foods and soap).
- Fresh leaf paste of fenugreek applied on face every night before going to bed and washed off wit warm water next morning.

13. Bleeding in nose, body heat

- Juice of fresh coriander leaves used as nasal drops.
- Lemon juice dropped into nostrils.

- Soak 8 to 10 almonds and 1 tsp rice overnight. Remove the outer skin. Grind into a fine paste. Mix in some milk and a pinch of turmeric powder. Boil and drink along with sugar candy.
- Take a tender fruit of Bel. Grind it in 1 teacup milk. Apply on head and massage well before showering off.
- Soak 1 tbsp turmeric bits in slaked lime for a couple of hours. Remove the bits. Dry them in the sun. Powder them. This rose-coloured powder can be preserved in a vial. Ten pinches of this powder are to be taken along with hot water, milk or honey. Twice daily.

14. Bleeding piles

- Take 1 tsp dried powder of peepul leaves with warm water.
- Take 1 tsp juice extracted from bittergourd leaves. Mix into a glassful of buttermilk and take every morning.
- Mix ½ tsp powder of mango kernel in a teacup of whey and drink.
- Take 1tsp of the inner bark of neem tree and mix it with 2 tsps of jaggery powder.
- Extract the juice from 1 cup tamarind leaves and apply on the affected parts.
- Half tsp each powder of dried pomegranate flowers, khuskhus and dried neem leaves, taken twice a day along with milk.

15. Blood Pressure

- For giddiness due to BP, Mix 1 tsp cardamom seeds with 2 tsp dried ginger, long pepper and liquorice. Powder it. Add 5 tbsp sugar. Take ½ tsp in a cup of hot water twice a day.
- Soak in a glass of water 1 tsp each coriander seeds, sandal paste and dried amla fruits. Strain and drink the water next morning.
- For high BP, Mix 1 tsp finely ground cumin power in 2 tbsp each coconut water and milk and ¼ tsp freshly ground sandal paste and sugar to taste. Drink this mixture every morning for a few days.
- Boil a tsp of garlic in 1 teacup milk. Take twice a day.
- For low BP, add ¾ teacup crushed liquorice root to 4 teacups cold water and allow it to stand for 2 hrs. Then bring it quickly

to a boil and steep for 5 mts. Add this to the bathwater in the tub. Take juice of tulsi leaves (10-15) mixed with 1 tsp honey.

16. Boils

- Tie a fresh thin banana leaf on the affected area.
- Dissolve 1 tbsp refined flour in a very little water. Heat 1 tsp coconut oil and fry the flour till it is softened. Spread it over a thin muslin cloth and apply on the boil when it is still bearably warm.

  Mash garlic cloves and apply externally.
- Apply a paste of ginger powder and turmeric (1:1) on boils.
- Boil 1 teacup water. Add 2 tsp ground mustard and 1 tsp sugar candy. Allow it to cool. An oil-spill-like-skin that appears on the surface is skimmed off and applied on the affected areas.
- Heat pepper powder in ½ tsp ghee until charred. Use this as ointment. (caution : pepper burns!)

17. Burning eyes

- Mash 1 ripe banana along with a little curd and water, take twice a day.
- Take a tender fruit of Bel. Grind it in 1 teacup milk. Apply on head and massage well before showering off.
- Grind an onion with 1 tsp each black pepper and ½ teacup khuskhus in milk. Apply this paste on the head.
- Mix the juice of bottlegourd and sesame oil (4:1) and heat till the moisture is evaporated completely. Once cool, use it for massaging the head.
- Mix equal quantities of fenugreek seed powder along with shikakai powder for washing hair. Wash frequently.

18. Burns

- Mash a ripe banana and apply on burns. Bandage with betel leaves.
- Apply curry leaves as poultices over affected areas.
- Combine 4 tsp each lime juice and coconut oil and rub until the mixture turns white. Apply on affected parts.
- Grind pomegranate flowers and apply the paste on affected parts.
- Make a paste of 1 tsp gel of aloe with 1 tsp turmeric powder and apply.

19. Cholesterol (high)

- Regular intake of coriander decoction made by boiling 2 tsp dry seed powder in 1 teacup water. (milk and sugar can be added to improve its taste. This could be a welcome substitute for tea or coffee). Note: This also acts as a diuretic as kidneys are stimulated.
- 2-3 raw carrots a day for several days.
- Regular intake of garlic cloves for a few days.
- Make a paste of 2 tbsp durva (doob) grass, 6 black peppercorns and 2 pinches of cumin. Take twice a day along with buttermilk or coconut water.
- Finely dice an onion and mix it with 1 cup buttermilk along with ¼ tsp pepper powder and drink.

20. Cold

- Extract 1 tsp each juice from fresh ginger, betel leaf and tulsi leaves. Add 1 tsp honey. Take 2 or 3 times a day.
- 2 garlic cloves crushed, boiled in a cup of water along with ½ tsp turmeric powder.
- Ginger pieces, boiled in a glass of water and taken after straining with ½ tsp sugar.
- Boil in 2 teacups water, 1 tbsp grated fresh ginger, 1 tsp cinnamon powder and 1 tsp liquorice. Take 1 cup of this decoction once every 3 hours, sweetened by 1 tsp honey.
- Boil 1 tbsp fresh ginger paste, 1 tsp each liquorice and cinnamon powder in 1 cup water for 10 mts. Add honey and drink.
- Crush 1 tbsp vasaka leaves and boil in 2 cups of water till reduced to 1 cup. Add 1 tsp honey. Drink ½ cup twice a day for 40 days.
- Squeeze one lemon in a glass of hot water and add 1 tsp honey and 2 tbsp brandy. Drink before retiring to bed.

21. Constipation

- Grind separately 5 tsp almonds and 5 tsp dried dates. Combine them and add 10 tsp honey. Take 3 tsp of this mixture twice daily.
- Soak 2-3 almonds and dried figs for a few hours in 1 teacup water. Remove the outer skin of the almonds and grind together to a paste. Add 1 tbsp honey and eat before going to bed.

- Eat 6 tsp gulkand with milk
- Regular intake of ripe bananas.
- Mix the pulp of a ripe Bel with jaggery and eat once a day.
- Soak 1 or 2 dried amla fruits in water overnight. Mash and filter the next morning. Add 1 tsp honey and drink.
- Make a very fine powder of one tsp each of the following: saunf, dried ginger, senna leaves and rock salt. Dose : 1tsp with water at bedtime.

22. Cough

- Mix ½ tsp ajwain seeds, 2 cloves and a pinch of salt. Powder and sip with a little warm water frequently.
- Add to 1 teacup boiling water ½ tsp each ground long pepper, cloves and rock salt, and let the mixture steep fro 10 minutes. Filter, and drink while still warm.
- Prepare a tea of ½ tsp ginger, with ¼ each cinnamon and cloves per cup of water. Sweeten with 1 tsp honey and drink.
- Add 1 to 3 drops saunf oil to 1 tbsp honey. Take one teaspoon at a time.
- For hoarseness, gargle with warm saturated solution of saunf water.
- Juice of tulsi leaves (10-15) with 1 tsp each juice of ginger, betel leaf and honey.
- Tulsi leaves (15-20), frequently chewed with jaggery.

23. Cramps (muscular)

- Apply clove oil as poultice on the affected parts.

24. Dandruff

- Mix equal quantities of dried curry leaves, lime peel, shikakai, fenugreek seeds and green gram and grind them finely. Store and use as a substitute for soap or shampoo.
- Grind an onion with 1 tsp each black pepper and ½ teacup khuskhus in milk. Apply this paste on the head.
- Grind 1 tbsp root pieces of liquorice in 1 teacup milk with ¼ tsp saffron. Apply this paste at bedtime continuously.
- A handful of neem leaves boiled in 4 teacups water. After cooling and filtering the decoction is used for rinsing hair.
- Grind the sesame leaves into a very fine paste. Apply on the scalp. After 10 mts., rinse.

25. Dehydration

- Add ¼ tsp salt, 3 tsp brown sugar and 2 tsp lime juice to 1 teacup of water, mix well and drink.
- Due to diarrhea, soak half a nutmeg in 2 teacups water for over 2-3 hours. Take 1 tsp of this infusion and mix in 1 teacup fresh coconut water. Drink twice or thrice a day.

26. Depression

- Boil ¼ tsp powdered seeds of cardamom in thin tea water and drink.
- Mix 1/8 tsp nutmeg powder with 1 tbsp freshly extracted amla juice. Take 3 times a day.

27. Diabetes

- Boil 1 tbsp powdered banyan bark in 2 cups water till the volume is reduced to ½ cup. Filter and drink.
- Soak 1 tbsp chips of the banyan bark overnight in a glass of water. Drink the infusion the next morning.
- Mix ¼ tsp asafetida powder in 2 tsp bitter gourd juice. Take twice a day.
- Frequent intake of carrot juice.
- Mix 2 tsp lime juice in 4 tsp amla juice and 1 tsp honey. Take in the morning on an empty stomach.
- Roast saunf slightly on a heated ladle. Powder, sieve and bottle. Take ½ tsp of this churan twice a day along with warm water.

28. Diarrhoea

- Mash 1 ripe banana along with a pinch of salt and 1 tsp tamarind pulp. Take twice a day.
- Take a small, tender budding bel fruit and grind it with 1 tbsp curd. Take 1 to 2 tsp.
- Boil ¼ tsp powdered cardamom seeds in thin tea water and drink.
- Combine 1 tsp each powdered ginger, cumin and cinnamon with honey and make into a thick paste. Take 1 tsp thrice daily.
- 2 or 3 tsp coriander seeds soaked overnight in water and taken next morning with 1 teacup buttermilk.
- Mix juice of 15-20 tender curry leaves with 1 tsp honey and drink.

29. Eyesight weakness

- Mix seeds of cardamom along with 1 tbsp honey. Eat everyday.
- Extract the pure sap of the cleaned Durva (Doob) grass and use as eye drops. (caution : Take all necessary precautions to prevent infection).
- Boil 1 cup fenugreek leaves and eat with honey. Twice daily.
- Juice of onion flowers, to be used as eye drops.
- Sliced onion shoots fried in ghee and eaten frequently. (Caution: This should not be given to children continuously.
- If there is strain on eyes due to watching TV and excessive reading habits, boil ½ tsp saunf in a cup of water till it is reduced to half. Cool. Use as eye drops (Caution: Beware of contamination).

30. Fatigue

- Fry in 1 tbsp ghee ½ tsp each coriander seeds, cumin seeds, black pepper, tail pepper and tuvar dal. Make a tasty rasam by adding 1 tsp rasam powder, one tomato and 1 teacup water. Drink it as an appetizer or eat with steamed rice.
- Add ¾ teacup crushed liquorice root to 4 teacups cold water and allow it to stand for 2 hrs. Then bring it quickly to a boil and steep for 5 mts. Ad this to the bathwater in the tub.
- Add to bathwater 4 teacups cold water in which 1 teacup mustard powder tied in a cloth bag had been steeped for 2-3 hrs.
- If there is exhaustion due to overwork, boil ¼ tsp powdered seeds of cardamom in thin tea water and drink.

31. Fever

- 1 tsp fresh ginger juice mixed with a cup of fenugreek decoction and 1 tsp honey.
- Extract 1 tsp each juice from tulsi leaves and bel flowers. Add 1 tsp honey. Take twice a day.
- Half tsp ground pepper is mixed in warm water along with 1 tsp palm candy. This drink is taken at bedtime.
- Add 1 tbsp leaves of pudina to 1 teacup water. Take twice or thrice a day.
- Clean, crush and boil a handful of mint leaves along with a paste made of ½ tsp black pepper, ½ tsp long pepper and 1 tsp

dry ginger power in 2 teacups water, till reduced to 1 teacup. Filter and divide into 3 equal doses and take 3 times a day.

- Boil 2 tbsp saunf in 1 teacup water till it is reduced to half. Filter. Take 1 tbsp every morning and evening for a few days. (This filtrate, when used to wash the eyes frequently, is reported to strengthen the eye muscles. It is a good cleansing lotion for inflamed eyes.)

32. Gum diseases

- If gums are bleeding, drink often lime juice in water. Simultaneously massage the gum frequently with coconut oil.
- In case of pus formation, a mixture of equal quantities of fine salt and pepper powder, thoroughly massaged over the gums.
- For dental problems, turmeric burnt, and finely powdered used as toothpowder.
- For gum inflammation, mix ½ tsp salt with 1 cup ginger water. Apply by dipping finger in water and rubbing on gums.
- Crush equal quantities of onions and onion flowers and extract the juice. Gargle frequently with this.

33. Hair loss

- Apply a little almond oil on scalp frequently and massage.
- Heat 10 flowers of Chinese hibiscus flowers in 2 teacups coconut oil till charred. Filter and use as hair oil.
- Massage with coconut oil everyday.
- Mix dried rind of lime, with shikakai, curry leaves, seeds of fenugreek and green gram- all in equal quantities. Powder it and use for washing hair.
- Grind 1 tbsp each pulp of amla with lime juice. Massage this into the hair before going to bed. Wash it next morning.

34. Headache

- Grind the fresh amla fruits into a fine paste and apply on affected parts.
- Use rose petals as a cold compress for the forehead.
- Mix finely powdered tail pepper and dried ginger (sonth) 1 tsp each in a little rose water and apply on the affected area.

- Apply the leaf-paste of henna on the affected parts.
- Grind a handful of henna leaves with 1 tbsp lime juice and apply on the affected parts.
- Make a smooth paste of cloves, water and salt. Apply on the affected areas.
- Mix equal quantities of sandal paste and coriander seed powder in an adequate quantity of water. Apply the paste on the affected areas.

35. Hiccups

- Take ½ tsp powder of black cumin seeds with a glass of buttermilk.
- Mix 2 tsp mustard powder in 1 teacup hot water. Sip.
- Mix 1/8 tsp nutmeg powder with 1 tbsp freshly extracted amla juice. Take 3 times a daily.
- Add 1 tbsp pudina leaves to 1 teacup water. Take twice or thrice a day.
- Add to 1 teacup boiling water ½ tsp each ground long pepper, cloves and rock salt, and let the mixture steep or 10 minutes. Filter, and drink while still warm.

36. Insect bites

- Drink 2 or 3 tsp coriander leaf juice mixed in 1 teacup water. Also apply sandalwood paste on the affected area.
- Mix the fruit pulp of curry leaf plant with an equal quantity of lime juice and apply on affected parts.
- Take 1 tsp leaf juice and drink with water. Also apply externally.
- Split the fresh leaves of Aloe and expose the fresh juice to the sun for a while and then rub on the affected parts.

37. Insomnia

- Steep 1 tbsp mint leaves in 1 teacup water for 30mts. Drink the infusion. Do not boil.
- Grind blanched almonds (8 to 10) along with 1 tsp khuskhus in ½ teacup milk and smear the paste on palms and soles at bedtime.
- Mix 1 tsp powder of fried cumin with a mashed ripe banana. Eat at night regularly.

- 2 tsp fresh juice of fenugreek leaves along with 1 tsp honey taken daily.
- Thoroughly mix rose oil (3 drops), violet oil (3 drops) and sweet almond oil (4 tbsp) and preserve. Apply to the scalp, ears and soles of the feet before sleeping. 1 tbsp each khuskhus and Cannabis leaves commonly used in the preparation of bhang are ground with a little water and applied on soles and palms before going to bed.
- Mix 1/8 tsp nutmeg powder with 1 tbsp freshly extracted amla juice. Take 3 times a daily.
- Boil a mixture of equal quantities of aloe leaf juice and gingelly oil till all moisture has evaporated. Apply on the head and massage for a few minutes before retiring.

38. Intestinal worms

- Burn some of the banana roots in the fire. Collect the ash. Take ¼ teaspoonful of this ash mixed with honey for a few days.
- Take 5-10 seeds of bitter gourd and crush them. Fry them in a little ghee. Take twice daily.
- 3-4 garlic cloves steeped in water or milk overnight; the liquid is drunk next day.
- Methi seeds, fried and powdered. This is added to drinking water. 2-3 times daily for 3-2 days.
- Fry 1 tsp dried neem flowers in 1 tsp ghee and mix with 1 teacup boiled rice and eat twice or thrice a day.

39. Jaundice

- Mash a ripe banana along with 1 tbsp honey and eat twice a day for a few days.
- Finely grind some bel leaves. Take 1 tsp of this paste along with a pinch of black pepper and follow with 1 teacup buttermilk thrice a day.
- ½ tsp ginger juice with 1 tsp each fresh lime and pudina juice mixed with a tbsp of honey, taken frequently.
- Soak overnight 1 tsp tamarind pulp along with 1 tbsp dried alubukhara (plums). Mash in the morning. Add a little black salt and eat.
- A fine paste of tender leaves of papaya (1/2 tsp) is taken with some water.

40. Lactation in mothers

- To increase lactation, ½ tsp finely ground cinnamon to be taken every night along with 1 teacup milk.
- Mix together 1 tsp each cumin power and sugar and take with warm milk after dinner every day for a few days.
- Mix ½ tsp powdered seeds of fenugreek along with dalia or rice porridge and eat daily.
- Eat cooked unripe fruits of papaya frequently.
- Boil 2 tsp saunf in barley water and take twice or thrice a day.

41. Leucorrhoea

- Boil 1 tsp saffron in ¼ teacup water. Let it reduce to become 1 tbsp. Divide this decoction into three portions and take with equal quantity of water, thrice daily for a couple of days.
- Mix 1 tsp leaf juice of Shatavari in a glass of milk and drink.
- Soak some crushed bark of peepul overnight in a mug of water and use it to douche the affected areas frequently.
- Cook a handful of Dronapushpi leaves along with greens and a little tamarind. Eat with chapattis or cooked rice.
- Boil 1 tbsp banyan bark in 2 cups water till the volume is reduced to ½ cup. Add ½ cup milk and 1 tsp palm sugar and drink. Once daily for 15 days.

42. Lumbago

- Take equal quantity of asparagus seeds (Shatavari), black cumin seeds, fenugreek seeds and ajwain. Powder. Take ½ tsp of this powder every morning.
- Mix mustard oil with rectified alcohol (1:40) and use as a lotion on affected parts.
- Mix ½ tsp root-milk powder of Ashwagandha with equal quantities of sugar, honey, powder of long pepper and ghee. Take once or twice a day.
- In case of lumbago pain accompanying menstruation, boil 1 tsp saffron in ¼ teacup water. Let it reduce to become 1 tbsp. Divide this decoction into three portions and take with equal quantity of water, thrice daily for a couple of days.
- Apply the sap of the banyan tree on the affected areas.

43. Memory improvement

- Mix 1 tsp each root powder of amla and white sesame seed powder. Add 1 tsp honey and eat everyday for a few days.
- Pluck 10 leaves of Brahmi and wash in hot water. Grind them with 5 black peppercorns. Mix into a glass of buttermilk and drink on an empty stomach every morning for 3 to 6 months.
- Take ½ tsp black cumin powder and mix it with honey. Eat small quantities twice a day.
- Take a mixture of 1 tsp honey and a pinch of finely powdered cinnamon every night regularly.

44. Mouth ulcers

- Mix 1 teacup pulp of Bel with 1 tsp sugar and eat early morning on an empty stomach for 3 days. Take 1 tsp finely powdered root bark of amla and mix with honey. Apply on affected areas frequently.
- Mix some coconut milk with honey and massage the gums 3 to 4 times a day.
- Coriander decoction prepared by boiling 1 tsp seeds in 1 teacup water, gargled when lukewarm, frequently.
- Methi seeds, fried and powdered. This is added to drinking water. 2-3 times daily for 2-3 days.
- Soak 1 tbsp crushed liquorice root in 2 teacups water for 2 to 3 hrs and use it for gargling frequently.

45. Muscular pain

- Soak ½ tsp liquorice root powder in 1 teacup water and leave overnight. Mix into the infusion 1 teacup rice gruel (cooked broken rice) and take every morning.
- Warm the papaya leaf over the fire and apply on affected parts.
- Heat ginger paste with turmeric paste (1:1) and apply.
- Boil 1 tbsp dried and powdered of Ashwagandha in 5 tbsp gingelly oil and apply on the affected parts when bearably hot.
- Take ¼ tsp Brahmi (powder of the dried leaves) along with honey or cow's milk or buttermilk.

46. Nervous Weakness

- Soak 8 to 10 almonds for a few hours and remove the outer skin. Grind the kernels along with 8 to 10 black peppercorns into a very thin paste. Mix into 1 teacup milk and take daily.

- Mix seeds of cardamom along with 1tbsp honey. Eat every day.
- Frequent intake of coriander tea: boil or steep 2 tsp coriander powder in a glass of water. Add sugar and milk to taste.
- Mix ½ tsp root milk powder of Ashwagandha along with 1 tbsp palm sugar, in 1 cup cow's milk. Take at bedtime.
- Take ¼ tsp Brahmi (powder of the dried leaves) along with honey or cow's milk or buttermilk.

47. Obesity

- Saunf tea could be an ideal medicine for obesity. Boil 1 tsp saunf in 1 cup toned milk for 5 to 10 minutes. Filter. Add sugar if necessary. Sip as hot as possible.
- Grind 6 to 7 blanched almonds, 1 tsp rice, 1 or 2 tbsp juice of banana flower into a fine paste. Pour into this some milk and drink everyday for 40 days.
- Eat 10 fresh, fully grown curry leave every morning for 3 to 4 months. Avoid fatty foods, sweets and alcohol.
- Roast saunf slightly on a heated ladle. Powder, sieve and bottle. Take ½ tsp of this churan twice a day along with warm water.
- Mix ½ tsp black pepper powder in 1 tsp honey and 3 tsp lime juice. Add 1 cup water and drink daily.

48. Phlegm

- Two garlic cloves curshed, boiled in a cup of water along with ½ tsp turmeric powder.
- Fry 1 tsp dried neem flowers in 1 tsp ghee and mix with 1teacup boiled rice and eat twice or thrice a day.
- Boil 2 tbsp saunf in 1 teacup water till it is reduced to half. Filter. Take 1 tbsp every morning and evening for a few days. (This filtrate, when used to wash the eyes frequently, is reported to strengthen the eye muscles. It is a good cleansing lotion for inflamed eyes).
- Heat 1 tsp garlic in 3 tbsp gingelly oil. Rub this preparation on the chest and throat.
- Finely powder the dried leaf of Basil (tulsi). Use as snuff.

49. Psoriasis

- Powder a few almonds and boil thoroughly in some water. Apply this paste on affected areas and let it remain overnight. Next morning wash it off with water.
- Lime juice, diluted in water and used as soap.
- Very thin slices of onions fried in ghee, eaten frequently. (Caution: Excess intake may cause coughing and gas in stomach).
- Boil 1 tsp sandalwood powder in 3 cups water till it is reduced to 1 cup. Add a little rose water and sugar and take thrice a day.
- Boil the Brahmi leaf juice in ghee and apply.

50. Sexual Debility

- Fry equal quantities of ajwain seeds and kernel of tamarind seeds in ghee. Powder and store in a dry, cool place. Mix 1 tsp of this powder in a glass of milk along with 1 tbsp honey. Drink daily at bedtime.
- Mix equal parts of rose hips and buds, tea leaves and jasmine flowers. Steep 2 tbsp of the mixture in 1 cup boiling water for 10 minutes. Sweeten with 1 tsp honey and drink.
- Soak 8 to 10 almonds for a few hours and remove the outer skin. Grind the kernels along with 8 to 10 black peppercorns into a very thin paste. Mix into 1 teacup milk and take daily.
- Fry a small piece of asafetida (1/4 tsp) in ghee. Add ½ tsp banyan latex. Eat in the morning every day along with a banana.
- Cut the stamens from 5 flowers of Chinese hibiscus and boil in a cup of milk and drink every day at bed time.

51. Tastelessness

- Boil 1 tsp mint leaves in 1 cup water. Take off the fire. Add ½ tsp powdered cardamom seeds, mix and drink (note - cardamom should never be boiled).
- Rub on the tongue a mixture of finely powdered cinnamon and honey and allow it to remain for sometime.
- Steep 1 tbsp mint leaves in 1 teacup water for 30mts. Drink the infusion. Do not boil.

- Clean and boil 1 tbsp root of Shatavari in a cup of milk. Strain, and add honey to improve the taste. Drink.
- Rasam, eitheras a drink or with plain, steamed rice.
  Rasam, the hot and tangy soup of southern cuisine can be used as a medicinal formulation, based on the permutation and combination of its constituent spices and condiments.

Step 1-grind the following - ½ tsp each cumin seeds, black pepper, coriander seeds, seedless tamarind pulp, curry leaves, garlic paste and ginger paste along with 1 ripe finely cut tomato and a little water. Boil well.

Step 2 : Fry ½ tsp mustard seeds along with a pinch of asafetida in 1 tsp ghee till it splutters. Add to the boiled mixture. Eat with plain steamed rice.

52. Toothache

- Burn the shells of almonds and powder. Use as toothpowder.
- Heat ½ tsp asafoetida in 2 tsp lime juice. Soak a piece of cotton in this solution and place it in the tooth cavity.
- Soak a piece of cotton wool in few drops of clove oil. Press on affected areas.
- Heat 1 tsp coconut oil and fry 3 pieces of clove. Powder. Apply on the affected areas.
- Paste of dry ginger applied to gums along with a little salt.
- A mixture of finely powdered pepper and clove oil is applied on the affected areas.

53. Tuberculosis

- Mix ripe banana along with ½ cup curd, 1 tsp honey and 1 teacup coconut water and take twice a day.
- In early states of TB, mix the pulp of the ripe bel fruit with required quantity of sugar and honey and take after dinner for 40 days.
- Half tsp garlic, boiled with 1 teacup milk and 4 teacups water, till reduced to one-fourth of the volume. The decoction to be taken thrice a day.
- Boil 20 leaves of basil (Tulsi) in 2 teacups water, reduced to 1 cup. Add to this 1 tsp sugar candy and 2 tsp honey. Take 2 tbsp two or three times a day.
- Take 10 to 20 drops of the leaf juice of Vasaka with 1 tsp honey thrice a day.

- Boil 2 teacups dried amla fruits in 4 teacups water till the volume is reduced to 1 teacup. In a separate vessel, make sugar syrup by dissolving 1 teacup sugar in adequate water and heating it. Now mix the amla decoction with sugar syrup and heat over a low flame and stir the mixture frequently. Separately mix the finely ground power of the following: 1 tbsp each dried ginger, black pepper and long pepper; 1 tbsp each cloves, cardamom, sal, (shorea robusta) liquorice, coriander seeds, cumin. Now, fold in the powder mixture little by little into the boiling mixture while stirring. Allow it to be heated till the desired consistency is obtained. Now add 1 tea cup of ghee made from cow's milk, stir will and remove from fire. Once the mixture is cooled, it can be stored in a clean, dry glass bottle. Take 1 tsp mixture along with a little milk twice a day.

54. Urinary diseases

- Mix 1 tbsp juice of amla with a ripe, mashed banana and eat twice or thrice a day.
- Soak 10 flowers of Chinese Hibiscus in a jug of water overnight and use this frequently for drinking.
- An infusion of tender leaves of papaya is taken once or twice a day.
- Juice of tulsi leaves (10-15) mixed with 1 tsp honey to be taken frequently.
- Boil ½ cup of clean Durva (doob) grass with an equal quantity of the tender leaves of pomegranate in 2 cups of water till reduced to 1 cup. Strain and cool. Dose: ½ cup. Repeat after two hours.

55. Wrinkles

- Apply coconut oil on the portions of skin and face where wrinkles set in and gently massage every night at bed time.
- Fresh leaf paste of fenugreek applied on face every night before going to bed and washed off with warm water next morning.
- Soak shredded ginger in honey. Eat a spoonful every morning.
- Split the fresh leaves of Aloe and expose the fresh juice to the sun for a while and then rub on the affected parts.
- Take ¼ tsp Brahmi (powder of the dried leaves) along with honey or cow's milk or buttermilk.

References

1. Aswal, B.S. et at. 1984. Screning of India plants for biological activity. Part XI.Indian J.Exptl.Biol. 22:487. (Pudina shows diuretic properties).
2. Bhat, J. V. and R.Broker. 1953. Action of some plant extracts on pathogenic Staphylococci. J. Sci. Industr. Res. 12:540-542. (Tulsi's anti-bacterial properties).
3. Chopra, R.N. et al 1958. Indigenous Drugs of India: Their Medical or Economic Aspects. Calcutta: U.N. Dhur & Sons. (Fenugreek as a component of home remedies).
4. Chopra, R.N. et al. 1956. Glossary of Indian Medicinal Plants. New Delhi: CSIR.7. (Use in rheumatism and bronchial asthma).
5. Dhew. 1974. A Barefoot Doctor's Manual. Publn. No. (NIH) 75-695, Washington D.C. (How coriander can be used as a household remedy).
6. Grover, G.S. and J.T. Rao. 1977. Investigations on the anti-microbial efficiency of essential oils from Ocimum sanctum and Ocimum gratissimum. Perfum. and Kosmef. 58(11):326-328. (Tulsi's essential oil exhibits anti-microbial effect; it was found active against fungi like Aspergillus niger, R. stolonifer and Penicillium digitatum).
7. Howes, F.N. 1949. Nuts: Their production and everyday uses. London: Faber & Faber. pp. 110-112.
8. Jain, M.P, 1983 . Vasaka, an Ayurvedic plant. Science Rep. 26(6): 350-357. (A survey of vasaka).
9. Khan, B. A. et al. 1995. Hypoglycemic action of Murraya Koenigii (Curry Leaf) and Brassica Juncea (Mustard): Mechanism of Action. Indian J. Biochem. Biophys. 32 (2):106.
10. Khandeparker, U.K. and R. Kulkarni. 1981. Anti-fatigue effect of Indigenous drug 'geriforte' in rats. Indian Drugs 18:346 (Nutmeg as a constitutent contributed to anti-fatigue property of the drug.
11. Kirtikar, K.R. and B.D. Basu. 1935. Indian Medicinal Plants. Revised By E.Blatter et al. 2nd edition. VoI. III. Allahabad. p. 2149. (Cinnamon as a medicinal plant).
12. Kureel, S.P. et al. 1970. Two novl alkaloids from Nurraya Koenigii Spreng. mahanimbicine and bicyclomahanimbicine. Chem. & Ind. 1950.
13. Lee, C.Y. et al. 1982. Study on the anti-oxidative activities of spices grown in Taiwan. Chung-kuo Nung Yeh Hua Hsues Hui Chih 20 (1-2):61; Chem. Abstr. 1982, 97, 143288p. (Anti-oxidative activities of ginger).

14. Nair, P.K. S. et al. 1987. Therapeutic effect of coconut shell extract in Dermatophytosis. J. Res. Ayur. Sid. VIII, 1&2:46-52. (Coconut exhibits a very significant anti-fungal activity).
15. Rai, A.N. et al. 1980. Effect of Yashtimadhu (Glycyrrhiza glabra Linn) on conjunctivitis. J. Res. Ayur. Sid. 1, 1:21-24. (Clinical parameters and microbiological studies confirmed the drug's efficacy particularly in acute conditions. Cortisone-like anti-inflammatory potential is also reported).
16. Ramesh Chandra. et al. 1978. A clinical trail of Gasex in gastro-intestinal symptoms. Probe 27 (4): 330-333. (2 tablets of Gasex, containing pudina, thrice daily was found effective in flatulence and abdominal discomfort, acidity and nausea).
17. Rao, A. et al. 1973. The effect of mandukaparni (Centella asiatica) on the general mental ability (Medhya) of mentally retarded children. J.Res. Indian Med. 8(4):9-15.
18. Roy, S.N. and S. Mukherji. 1979. Influence of food tannin on certain aspects of iron metabolism. Part III. Indian J. Biochem. Biophys. 16: 151. (Tannin from green bananas might aid in iron utilization in anaemia).
19. Sanyal, A.K. et al. 1961. Banana and gastric ulcer. (Letters to the editor) J. Pharm. Pharmacol. 13:318. (Banana in the treatment of gastric ulcers).
20. Shankaracharya, N.B. and C.P. Natarajan. 1971. Coriander Chemistry, Technology and Uses. Indian Spices Vol. 8(2) p. 4.
21. Sharma, R. et al. 1987. Efficacy of Bacopa minnieri in revitalizing intellectual functions in children. Jour. Res. Edn. Ind. med. 6(1-2):1-10. (Revitalizes the intellect).
22. Singh, R.H. et al. 1981. Psychotropic effect of Medhya Rasayana drug Mandukaparni (Hydrocotyle asiatica). Part III, J. Res. Ayur. Sidha 2(1):110. (Cure for anxiety-neurosis).
23. Tanaka, T.E. 1976. Tanaka's Cyclopaedia of Edible Plants of the World. E. S. Nakro. Tokyo: Keigaku Publishing Co. (Lime: Properties and uses).
24. Tonnesen HH: From Chemistry on Curcumin and Curcuminnoids In Phenolic compounds in food and their effect on health Volume 1: Analysis, Occurrence and Chemistry. ACS Symposium Series no. 506 edited by Ho CT, Lee CY -Huant MT. Washington, DC: American Chemical Society, 1992, 143-153.

25. Watt, J.M. and M.G. Breyer-Brandwijk. 1962. The Medicinal and Poisonous Plants of Southern and Eastern Africa. 2nd edition. Edinburgh. p. 531. (Curativ properties of cinnamon).

26. Winton, A.L. and K.B.Winton. 1935. The Structure and composition of Foods. Wiley, 1:480-485. (Nutritive wealth of almond).

31

Newly Married Women – Some Advice on Demedicalised Approach to Life

Samiksha Singh

Young married couples are group of people who have not received the attention they deserve from the health care planners in India. They are the people who have entered that phase of life where they will soon be playing the role of parents; Investing in their well-being is important to make sure that young people enter adulthood with appropriate knowledge and accurate information about sexual, reproductive and general health to become responsible parents.

Surveys and research in India still find evidence of early marriages,[1] before the age of 20, with their accompanying poor pregnancy and birth outcomes. Our culture places significant pressure on newly married couples to quickly have their first child in order to confirm their fertility thus the use of contraception before the first child is strongly discouraged by both parents and in-laws.[2] The negative physical, social and psychological consequences of early marriage and childbearing for these young couples, their children and society make it essential to address the issue in depth and provide appropriate intervention for prevention of the same.

Not all young people have a clear understanding of what the concept of reproductive health entails. They do not understand the physiology of reproduction of males and females and other topics related to marital, reproductive and sexual health. They could have heard of issues but they are not necessarily well informed. The Engaged and newly married couples often know very little or have incorrect information about fertility, contraception and sexually transmitted diseases. They have significant information needs. Furthermore, as a result of the social taboos around the discussion of sex, these couples may have misconceptions about their bodies and about ways to achieve sexual satisfaction with their spouses.[3,4]

A USAID funded, TAHSEEN Project, on young, engaged and newly married people of Egypt, has documented that newly married females list a number of topics that they feel are important for women to know even before marriage. These include: sexual intercourse; sexual relationships; related hygiene; developing mutual understanding and consideration; dealing with sexual embarrassment and nervousness between partners; procedures and benefits of premarital examinations, and family planning. Newly married males recommend a number of specific topics, including: STDs and how to avoid them; awareness of sexual health; disadvantages of early pregnancies; reproductive and psychological health of women; healthy sexual intercourse; and premarital examinations.[5]

More than half of the newly married women in India are adolescent women.[1] This group of young women receive very little guidance from their parents, school curricula or the media about gender roles and responsibilities, child bearing and rearing and similar issues to prepare them for their new life as wives. In this young age the women are not aware of the issues related to their reproductive health and family welfare. They also are not aware of their rights. So they fail to exercise them. They do not utilize health facilities to the desired extent. By the time they realize their needs; they have had many children and faced many gynecological and obstetric problems. Conventionally, the husband is expected to look after his wife as per our culture, and then it is appropriate that one of the important responsibilities of the husband after marriage is to ensure good health of his wife. First, the wife should be physically healthy. If there is any physical health problem then it should be sorted before the cycle of child bearing and/or rearing starts. If there is any pre-existing disease, it should be treated.

Health of newly married women

Marriage at right age, harmonious relationship with the spouse, equal status of women in decision making, appropriate planning and time of child birth, and access to health care-including counseling and supportive services - constitute the favourable atmosphere for health of married women. The marriage in itself is no determinant of ill health. It is the socio-cultural and psychosomatic issues attached to it which determine the health status of the newly married women.

As per our culture, when a newly wed woman shifts to the husband's house, she moves into an unknown environment with many apprehensions and expectations. It heavily depends on how much she is ready to accept and adjust and how she is welcome in the new family to help her settle faster and comfortably. The new relationships and the responsibilities attached to them may add some psychological stress. She is new in the environment and even for small decisions and facilities she depends on the husband and in-laws. If the environment is not conducive she may not even be able to express herself. This restricts her freedom to ask for and access any kind of care.

Apart from the relationships and role with the members of the new family she begins her sexual and family life mostly after marriage. Many of them feel stress in sexual relationship. Many might surrender out of fear, or are manipulated or forced into it. The unaware and underpowered women are vulnerable to unsafe sex, RTI/STIs and even sexual abuse.[6] The females who have optimal knowledge on reproductive health before marriage are better equipped to handle the inherent vulnerabilities of a woman in traditional sexual milieu – and enter into a healthy reproductive life.

Those young men and women who are unaware of the physiological and biological changes which may occur in the process and the diseases they might, if they, acquire, may develop unreasonable fears and discomfort in their relationships. It is needed that they understand these changes and about the ways to prevent several psychological and medical problems. They should be able to self diagnose the disease states and should know where and how to access the health care.

The newly married woman needs to be more vocal about her issues of concern to the husband and in-laws. She should be able to freely express her needs, and problems. She should have a say in decision making about sexuality, family planning and other issues in the family. She should be empowered enough to decide for herself and access health care whenever needed. She should be knowledgeable enough to take care of herself. She should be aware and skilled enough to be a healthy reproductive partner and a responsible parent.

The healthy, appropriately aware and responsive individuals will grow into responsible partners and parents. These individuals only may be able to experience sexual, reproductive and family health status of higher standards.

Newly married women should be educated on the following topics regarding health:

- Suitable age for a healthy marriage and pregnancy and health effects of early pregnancies on mother and child.
- General health of a women and Self care
- Value and importance of premarital examinations.
- The reproductive physiology of males and females.[7]
- Healthy and unhealthy sexual practices.
- STDs and their prevention.
- Communication within the couple.
- Importance of family planning and the use of contraceptives.
- Peri-conception health.
- Antenatal care and the importance of follow-up medical visit. (refer to other chapters)
- Exclusive breastfeeding and its importance for the health of the mother and child. (refer to other chapters)
- Child rearing issues (refer to other chapters)

Age for a healthy marriage and pregnancy

As per Indian law a female should be married after she has completed 18 yrs of age. Apart from legal issues, biologically and physiologically the female is immature to be a wife and lead her sexual and family life before attaining the age of 18 yrs. Studies show that, she should be at least 20 yrs old before conceiving and giving birth to a child. Even if the marriage has occurred earlier the first pregnancy should be postponed till after 20 years of age.

Health consequences of early marriage and early child birth:

If married early the girls are not able to complete their studies- They become dependent as well as vulnerable to harassment by in-laws and lack any power to decide for themselves. They are subjected to sexual abuse and forced into unhealthy sex. They may also have to suffer from various psychological and gynecological health problems.

Early child-bearing also leads to several complications. Among the health consequences of early childbearing are, for the woman, higher than average levels of blood pressure, toxaemia, anaemia, bleeding, obstructed and difficult labour, premature delivery and death. In addition, children born to teenage mothers are susceptible to higher incidence of low birth weight, prematurity, still birth and perinatal mortality.[8] Child birth by women at the age of 20-25 yrs is known to have reported least complications to both mother and child.[9,10]

Premarital examinations

This is not a common practice in our community. The youth should know about the identification of hereditary problems through premarital examinations and blood group differences. Hereditary diseases are commoner in marriages among blood relatives. A few important infectious diseases like HIV/AIDS can be and should be diagnosed before entering into marriage alliance. These may harm the other partner and also the offspring. They should understand that early detection of health problems prevents jeopardizing one's marriage later on.

Hereditary diseases are carried in human genes. The interaction of genes from mother and father determine the occurrence or absence of the disease. Genes are always in pairs. One or both members of the pair may be dominant or recessive. Not all hereditary diseases manifest in the individual. Those manifesting may be characterized by dominant genes, i.e. if even a single dominant gene carrying the disease characteristics is present in the pair of gene in the individual then disease may manifest its signs and symptoms. Thus, if the disease carrying genes are dominant it will manifest in both homozygous (both genes in the pair are similar and dominant) as well as heterozygous (genes in the pair are not similar; one is dominant and the other is recessive) condition. If the disease carrying genes are recessive, the disease manifests in homozygous condition only (both genes in the pair are recessive). In heterozygous condition the normal dominant gene suppresses the disease carrying recessive disease. Such individuals are symptomless and remain undiagnosed despite their passing the disease carrying gene. But they have potential to transmit this gene to the next generation. It is this undiagnosed disease group which needs to be identified before marriage. They are known as carriers. Both the male and female may look healthy and may be carrying one recessive gene. In such cases, the chances of giving birth to a diseased baby with both the recessive genes are 25% when a heterozygous male marries a heterozygous female. Many of such diseases are fatal eg. Thalassemia. Some such diseases may be carried by sex chromosomes eg. Haemophilia. Many such recessive diseases may not manifest in the mother but may manifest in male child. There are a number of hereditary diseases if diagnosed can be prevented by avoiding such marriages. [11]

Premarital medical examination is mandatory in some countries, like China.[12] Statistics from Beijing Public Health Bureau reveals that, from 1996 to 2002, a total of 15,794 people were found to have heredity diseases during premarital check-up. Among them, 695 were diagnosed as "not suitable to have children".

Premarital examinations should include the following: detailed history about the individual's past and present health status, history of any familial diseases in the family, complete physical examination, a total blood picture including hemoglobin analysis and bleeding and clotting time; Rh factor analysis; blood analysis for STDs (syphilis, AIDS) and hepatitis B & C; urine analysis for diabetes, Urinary tract infections and chronic renal failure; semen analysis, and chest X-ray. Other components included as part of premarital examinations are: analysis for toxoplasmosis, menstrual history, internal check, stool analysis and virus and hereditary disease analysis. The physicians should utilize this opportunity to offer counseling on such topics as overall health, the sexual relationship, interpersonal relations, role responsibilities and childbearing issues as an essential aspect of health consultation.

The decision to marry after knowing the existing medical problems in the marriage is the individual's own. If they proceed with such marriages they know the unknown and are prepared for the consequences. They can plan their life to prevent acquiring the disease themselves or transmitting the diseases to the next generation. Some of these examinations can be and should be done any time before planning the first child to rule out the possibility of transmitting common congenital infections and hereditary diseases to the child.

General health of women and self care:

One's own general health status is important for every human being irrespective of age, gender and social class. Good healthy status reflects into individual's harmonious state of mind and efficient work. To stay healthy is every individual's right. The adults capable of taking care of self should do so. In general the individual should take care of his nutrition, hygiene, regular physical exercise and other disease preventive and health promoting actions. Many of such issues for women in general have been discussed in other chapters.

For newly married, the general health issues are not different from those for other women. Few domains like promotion of menstrual and sexual hygiene, prevention and treatment of anaemia, reproductive tract infections and health during pregnancy are specifically described below for the newly married as they are to begin their sexual and family life. They may be at higher and immediate risk of acquiring RTIs and other diseases related to above mentioned domains.

Sexual Health

Sexual health requires a positive and respectful approach to sexuality and sexual relationships, as well as the possibility of having pleasurable and safe sexual experiences, free of coercion, discrimination and violence. For sexual health to be attained and maintained, the sexual rights of all persons must be respected, protected and fulfilled. This include the right to – the highest attainable standard of sexual health including access to sexual and reproductive health care services as well as information related to sexuality; sexuality education; respect for one's own and partner's bodily integrity; choose their partner; decide to be sexually active or not; consensual sexual relations; consensual marriage; decide whether or not, and when, to have children; and pursue a satisfying, safe and pleasurable sexual life.[13]

The above stated are the rights of every individual both male and female. In our society where talking about sex is a taboo, the newly married girls in particular are not expected to talk about the sexuality however they are expected to know their role in consummation of marriage, how to accept it with honour and dignity and simultaneously respect the spouse's needs and desires. It is reported that many newly married women do not know about sexual activity before marriage. At initiation of sexual alliance few surrender as they are told, else the husband may move to other women. Other few are tricked into it as they do not understand what it really means and many are forced by in-laws to do so.[14] These problems are faced more by the young newly married due to ignorance. Lack of the power to say no is a major factor in whatever is wrong with sexual relationships between newly married couples in India.

Also, most of the marriages in India are arranged. This does not give much opportunity to the couple to interact and develop a comfort level and liking for each other before marriage. Some married women in beginning of their marriage hate to be initiated into sexual activity but have no choice. This leads to discomfort in their relationships and often lead to violence and sexual abuse. Many women unaware of their sexual roles and rights fail to express their needs to their sex partners. They have many myths and misconceptions about their bodies. They fail to experience the pleasure of sexual activity. During our study on newly married women[14]- one of the participants asked the interviewer that "during the sexual act my husband feels excitation and pleasure but I do not feel anything. Is their any thing wrong with me?" Another participant was worried that she had discharge per-vagina during the sexual activity and she felt embarrassed. She was suspecting some disease in her body but was not able to talk about it to anyone.

Another hindrance to healthy and pleasurable sexual life is lack of communication on such issues within the marriage. Most women fail to express their needs, desires and apprehensions about sex and thus experience dissatisfaction and distress. A proper understanding of their roles and responsibilities can bring harmony in their married life. For healthy and pleasurable sexual activity:

- The young newly married women need to know and understand their and the men's reproductive and sexual physiology.
- Consummation of marriage is an essential component of successful marriage and the females should mentally prepare themselves for it. They should understand that it's a respectful and genuinely loving act if carried with mutual consensus.
- Both the partners should respect others needs and desires regarding sexuality. They need to work together towards integration of sexuality into mutually satisfying relationship.
- Women should permit the sexual relationship only when they are mentally and physically prepared for it else they may not experience pleasure, in fact they may even have to bear pain and injury if forced by the husband.
- Women should be vocal about their apprehensions and fears. Talking to the husband about sex may help them understand and accept it better. It may improve their performance, will avoid embarrassments and help them understand what excites and gives sexual pleasure to them. What works for both of them to experience the highest level of satisfaction needs to be individually explored by couples themselves.
- The conditions of the female orgasm depend upon the state of the mind just as much as in the case of the husband. The male, however, being more sensual, is more quickly aroused. Female is far less often ready for sex. In her unexcited state the vagina is lax, its walls are closed together, and their surfaces covered by little lubricating secretion. This may lead to inhibited painful experience. Once the female is comfortable and aroused the secretions in vagina will increase and it opens up to allow easier and comfortable entry.
- During initial sexual intercourse acts, it might not be very pleasurable, might be painful and may slightly bleed too. But in subsequent acts it improves and becomes easier and pleasurable.
- Seek medical care if any problem is faced.

Safe sex

It allows the couple to experience healthy pleasurable sexual life with mutual consensus without injuries, free of sexually transmitted infections including HIV/AIDS, without fear of having unintended pregnancy and avoiding unnatural and harmful forms of sex.

It is noted that the sex inside marriages is often unsafe for young females. This is because young females are more susceptible to sexually transmitted infections(STIs)[15], the frequency of sexual activity is more in the earlier married life, they are often married to older sexually experienced men who may be infected and condoms are used less within marriage than outside marriage.

To practice safe sex-

- Be faithful to your partner. Have sexual relationship with your spouse only.
- Have sexual activity with mutual consensus free of sexual abuse and coercion.
- Use contraceptive measures to prevent unwanted pregnancy.
- Use condoms with each sexual act to avoid STIs including HIV/AIDS and also unintended pregnancy.
- Practice adequate sexual hygiene.
- Avoid unnatural and harmful forms of sex.
- If any of the partners having any signs and symptoms of RTI/STI, then seek medical care and take complete treatment.

Reproductive tract infections / Sexually transmitted diseases

Reproductive tract infections are the group of infections of reproductive tract which may or may not (e.g. tuberculosis of uterus and adenexa), transmit through sexual contact. Sexually transmitted diseases are recognized as diseases which are transmitted through sexual contact but may or may not (e.g. HIV), cause reproductive tract infections. There are various micro-organisms which belong to both the groups and cause RTI/STDs diseases e.g. Gonorrhoea, Syphillis, Candida, Lymphogranuloma venerum etc.

STDs can be prevented from being transmitted from one to other by practicing safe sex and proper sex hygiene habits. This may reduce the probability of occurrence of many RTIs and will also prevent the spread of deadly HIV/AIDS.

RTIs if left untreated may lead to various complications like infertility through blocked fallopian tubes, ectopic gestation, pelvic inflammatory disease, vulval and cervical cancer, insanity and death. If the RTI is present during antenatal period, it may lead to trans-placental and peri-natal transmission to the baby in the womb. This can cause intra-uterine death, abnormal fetus, neonatal ophthalmic and ear infections as well as pneumonia. HIV infection and other STDs may also spread to the newborn in the antenatal or perinatal period and may cause AIDS early in childhood. RTIs can be prevented by preventing sexual transmission of infections. If RTIs have occurred then these can be self diagnosed at an early stage. Treatment early in time can prevent complications.

Characteristics of people having RTIs/STDs

Higher proportion of these infections in general population is seen in those sexually active young men and women who have -

- multiple sexual partners
- poor sexual hygiene
- poor menstrual hygiene in women

Some strata of population report higher rate of these infections eg. prostitutes, their clients, truck drivers, drug abusers, and refugees etc.[16]

RTIs/STDs in newly married women

It has been reported in various studies that young females have greater predisposition to acquiring RTIs/STIs. Their vagina is less acidic and the lining of the reproductive tract is not mature enough to fight these infections. In India, most of the females marry while in their adolescence thus their chances of acquiring RTIs/STIs is more than the women marrying at a later age. It is also seen that the infection is more common in the married than unmarried females. This can be thankfully attributed to conservative society in India that morally and socially restricts being sexually active before marriage. Immediately after marriage the young women become sexually active and the frequency of sexual contact is more than the older married women thus the young married women are at the highest risk of acquiring RTI/STIs.

It is important to address the issue early in the married life because if the RTI/STI occur in women and is left untreated, it may affect the women's fertility or health of the fetus if they successfully conceive.

Prevention and control of RTIs/STIs

* *Menstrual hygiene:*

- Use clean sanitary napkins/pads.
- If using cotton cloth avoid reuse of the same.
- If have to reuse the cloth wash it with soap and warm water and dry in sun.
- Irrespective of flow of blood in menses, change pads at least 2-3 times in a day.
- Change the soiled lingerie and cloths frequently.
- Wash genitals with potassium permanganate or soap and water.

• *Sexual hygiene:*

- Wash the genitals with soap and water before and after sexual contact.
- Douching of vagina with water and any antiseptic periodically is advisable
- Use condoms during every sexual act.
- Avoid unnatural forms of sex.
- Positively wash genitals before and after if having sex during menstruation phase.

• *Early self diagnosis of RTIs / STIs:*

• *Common signs and symptoms of RTIs in women* [17]

- White purulent/ curdy and / or foul smelling discharge from vagina.
- Pain in lower abdomen and lower back.
- Swelling in inguinal region.
- Ulcers in vulval region
- Itching in vulval region
- Burning micturition.

• *Common signs and symptoms of RTIs in men*

- White purulent/ curdy and / or foul smelling discharge from urethra.
- Swelling, redness and or pain in scrotum.
- Swelling in inguinal region.
- Ulcers over penis and surrounding area.
- Burning micturition.

Seeking health care and complete treatment:

If any of the above signs are detected the couple should seek medical treatment. The RTI/STIs are treatable. To avoid long term complications early treatment should be started for both the partners and complete treatment should be taken. Both the partners need to be treated simultaneously otherwise the untreated infective partner may re-infect the treated partner. The couple may be needed to undergo some blood and urine tests for confirmation of the disease agent. Where facility for lab diagnosis is not feasible the diagnosis can be made by the physician using the syndromic approach and treated accordingly. The infection still is completely treated. The couple should use condoms during each sexual act to prevent transmission of infection to one another. They should maintain healthy sexual hygiene.

Many women do not talk about these symptoms to anyone as they feel embarrassed and shy.[18,19] They often do not seek health care services as they are not allowed to by the husband and in-laws.[20] They should understand the seriousness of the RTI/STIs and that they must get treated to avoid later complications like PID, infertility, spontaneous abortion, ectopic pregnancy and cervical cancer etc. The female should talk about these to her husband or mother in-law without feeling embarrassed. They should themselves seek health care or request the husband and in-laws to help her get to medical facility in time. There should not be any taboo attached to it. The RTI/STIs are common in both men and women everywhere and most of them are absolutely treatable.

Treatment facilities for them are available in any of the government facilities; urban health centers and in rural primary health centers and above. Women can approach any of the near by facility for the treatment and referral if required. They should not feel shy to talk to the health professionals. The health care providers address such patients daily and can give the patient a much needed treatment advice in the right time.

Communication between husband and wife

Communication between the spouses is the key for a successful, harmonious and happy married life. The two will better understand each others' personalities, thoughts, desires, needs and problems if communication between them is proper. This is a first step towards building comfort and liking for each other. Healthy communication gives opportunity to discuss important issues. It aids in identifying mutual interests and issues of concern. This may also give opportunity to woman to present her view about family matters and have a role in decision making. Often the communication gap is a hindrance in attaining equal status for women in the family. Good communication builds up good relationship and confidence in the spouse. It creates a favorable environment for the woman to share her apprehensions and problems with the husband. This enables the couple to protect themselves, avoid harmful practices and address problems by seeking early diagnosis and treatment before complications arise.

Certain important issues are needed to be talked about early in a marriage. Issues like; conduct in the family, respect and care of self and other family members, sexuality, sexual hygiene, condom use, problems related to sex and STDs, family planning etc. Women should decide for herself first when to have a first child and convey her opinion to the husband. Final combined decision should be taken keeping in mind the interests of the wife the husband and the offspring to be born. As stated above, for child bearing, age less than 20 yrs of the women is not in favour of the mother or the child. The psycho-social and medical problems of the couple should also be talked about and investigated into before planning the first child.

The newly married female should not shy over these issues while talking to the husband. She should realize that it is important and it is her right as well as duty to do so for building a healthier relationship. If initiated by the husband she should respectfully accept and encourage such talks. This will help her to present her concerns also. And in case the talk is not initiated by the husband then she can start with general issues like conduct with other family members, to reduce the communication gap and build up comfort between the two. Once such comfort and faith builds in a relationship then it becomes easier to talk about much more sensitive issues. She should remember that without effective communication it is difficult to establish her suitable position in the family.

It is realized that overall family and reproductive health of women and men can not be achieved without each others support.

As in most instances the decision makers are males it becomes important to involve them even for reproductive health issues of women and family planning. This can be only achieved by making them aware of women's health and their role in achieving the higher standards of health status. Apart from the community based interventions to involve and educate men the wives should contribute in doing the same at their own family level as it is there where we need the men to responsibly take care of self and the wife's reproductive health; beginning from safe sex to taking care of pregnant wife to responsibly rearing the offspring and more.

Although in our conservative society the decision makers are mothers in laws in many cases but the scenario is changing with changing family dynamics, increasing education levels and working status of men and women. The communication in between the husband and wife will certainly show positive results in either case and promote role of women in decision making.[21,22]

Family planning and use of contraceptives[23]

It is advisable that the conception should be planned at least after one year of marriage. This is particularly applicable where the wife's age is less than 20-22 yrs. at marriage. However, this advice does not apply for women who marry late i.e. after 25 yrs. In such cases conception should be as early as possible after marriage. Overall, the decision should rest with the individual couples. It should be based on individual circumstances. In our society most of the marriages are arranged by the families. The couple does not get time to know and understand each other. Immediately after marriage they begin to adjust to the changed environment. More so for the wife as our culture requires her to leave her home and settle into the husband's home. She needs more time to get acquainted with the new relationships, new responsibilities and the new opportunities. It is needed that she psychologically and socially settles comfortably in the family. The wife and the husband should understand their roles and responsibilities before taking up a bigger responsibility of bearing and rearing a child. They should prepare themselves mentally, physiologically, socially and economically to bear a new responsibility which may bring along with it many of its needs. The first child should always be a planned child at the time most suitable to the couple. This will enhance the joy of the whole event.

What to use to postpone the first child birth?

Nowadays, many contraceptive choices are available for newly married women which do not cause much side effects and the fertility is resumed easily whenever the couple decides to conceive. The contraceptives preferred for newly married are:

1.Condoms: Condoms are preferred for newly married and young couples as it has dual protection; against pregnancy as well as sexually transmitted infections. They do not have any side effects except a few men reporting reaction to latex of condoms. If used appropriately with each sexual act they give good protection. The failure of protection occurs due to improper use, tear and spillage. Male condoms are applied during the sexual act on the erect penis of the males before penetrating into the female's vagina. The procedure and unwinding of the condom over the penis is pictorially shown over each condom pack. After that particular act the penis with the condom on should be withdrawn from the vagina avoiding spillage and then the condom should be removed and discarded. It should not be used again. Many couples initially complain of interference with sex. But, once the couple get used to it they have less complaints. It is the safest method available. In government health facilities condoms are available for free by the name of *Nirodh* even at the health centers in both urban and rural areas. Many more condom types with better qualities are available in market by various companies. These are often available at chemists and general stores.

2. Oral Contraceptive pills: They are of various types and should be used after taking the health care providers advice only.

3. Post coitus contraception / emergency contraception: If the newly married couple has had unprotected sex and fear to conceive then they may take emergency contraception within 72 hours of unprotected sex.

4. Coitus interruptus is a method wherein the male withdraws his penis out of the vagina before he is about to ejaculate. This prevents the entering of male's semen into the female's reproductive system and prevents conception. It is easier said than done and can have high failure rates.

5. Rhythm method or safe period method: This method is useful for the women having regular cycles i.e., they have menstruation at fixed dates of the month or up to plus minus 4-5 days. In woman's monthly menstrual cycle there are days (safe period) when if she has sex than the chances of getting pregnant are the least or conversely there are days (fertile period) when the woman if has sex than her chances of getting pregnant are more. For determining this subtract 18 from the shortest period of your cycle, this is the first day of the fertile period. Then subtract 10 from the longest period of the cycle, this gives the last period of the cycle. For example if the woman's cycle varies from 26-34 days then 8th (26-18=8) to 24th (34-10=24) day of the cycle is the fertile period to conceive and the remaining days are the safe period to have sex and not conceive. The first day is counted on the first day of menstrual bleeding. Other methods include abstinence which practically not possible in young married couples; basal body temperature method and cervical mucus method. These need correct knowledge and experience and they have higher failure rates.

After stopping contraceptive use when is one ready to conceive again?

If using condoms and natural methods, then one can conceive immediately after stopping their usage. In case of oral contraceptive pills it depends on the duration of their usage. If consumed for shorter period than fertility return within one or two cycles. If consumed oral pills for longer duration than it may take little more than two cycles. But return of normal cycles is almost always present after stopping any of the above temporary methods of contraception.

Why to have small families and when to plan second child?

The couple should plan for a small family consisting of not more than two children. And the second child should be planned at least after 2-3 years of the first child. Early planning may help cope with the future better. Small family and adequate spacing in between the two children is essential for the health of the mother and the children.

The women with many children are known to experience poorer health status specially those belonging to poorer socio-economic class. With each pregnancy they bear the risk to their health increases in that pregnancy. They may have more chances of hypertension, seizures, anaemia, metabolic disorders and retarded fetus. Many suffer with anaemia and other problems even after the pregnancy is over. It is seen that the later children of the multiparous women are born weak and that too with more chances of having congenital diseases. The children born to the women with age more than 30 years are more likely to have congenital disorders like Down's syndrome. Besides the direct effect on health of child many indirect factors lead to deterioration of health of the child. The more the number of children the more difficult is to keep account of their health status regularly. The available facilities as per the status of the parents get divided into several portions and none of the offsprings may get the minimal essential nutrition and other facilities. Often the children are neglected and their nutrition and immunizations are compromised. Later in life they may even be deprived of adequate education and psychological support. More number of children may add to psychological, social and economic burden on the family. Having small families is a responsible decision of the parents for their own health and the health of their children.

It is also important that there should be adequate, 2-3 years, interval in between two child births. It is shown in scientific research that after every child birth the female's body is in little deprived state and is not fit to bear another child. With good nutrition and health care her body takes 2-3 years to completely recover to normal healthy state to bear another child. If the child births occur more frequently her health state may continuously deteriorate without getting a chance to recover and likelihood of complications in the subsequent pregnancies will also increase. For the child: poorer the health status of the mother bearing the child poorer the health status of the newborn child. When a new baby is borne and the previous baby still very small and being breastfed the health of the earlier may be affected too. He will be deprived of the mother's attention, affection and breast milk much before he can afford too. This may lead to some negligence and negatively affect the health of the former child too.

It is necessary for the newly married couple to understand the importance of small family and adequate spacing between the two children. They should realize it to be important to decide this in the beginning and plan and act accordingly before unknowingly and unthoughtfully getting into state of no return. Early planning is required to avoid getting into a state of helplessness and regret.

What should be used for spacing between two children?

Apart from the above mentioned options the female have other options like Cu-T insertion and hormonal depot injections. The decision of what option to be used depends on the duration since last child birth, health status of the mother, lactating status, and menstrual status of the women. The advice should be sought from a doctor to decide when and what to use.

Peri-conception health:

We take care of the female to grow into a healthy woman to bear a healthy child and then we take care that during her pregnancy she stays in good health to give birth to a healthy child. But we forget about the time when she actually conceives and the first three months of pregnancy. At the time of conception the zygote is implanted into the mother's uterus and develops into an embryo. In the initial 3 months of conception the embryo develops into foetus and his various organ systems develop during this time. If the mother is healthy and takes required care then the whole process is healthy and the zygote develops into a healthy foetus. But the issue is that if the pregnancy is unplanned then this time period goes uncared for. Most of the women confirm their pregnancy status after 2 months and visit the health facility after 3-4 months. By this time the organ systems of the foetus have already taken basic shape and in the remaining time of pregnancy they just grow into mature systems. This is a domain which is usually neglected and there is no consideration towards working for healthy conception and healthy early antenatal period which is a very crucial period. Unless the couple has planned for the conception and is aware of the things to be taken care of in peri-conception period, the health care for the mother and the foetus cannot be provided during that period. Various attempts are being made all over the world to develop models for care of the couple in the peri-conception period for promoting healthy conception.[24] For this chapter we define peri-conception period as the time since the time of the planned conception to three months after conception. Important things to be taken care of in this period are:

1. Couple should always plan their child.
2. Both the parents should undergo preliminary pre-conception health check up before going for pregnancy at least for the

first baby. This is to rule out diseases of mother which put her and the child's health in danger and any risk of congenital infections or hereditary diseases to the child.

3. If mother is known to or diagnosed to have any medical problems like anaemia, jaundice, thyroid problems, diabetes, hypertension or any infections that may complicate pregnancy, then first she should get adequate treatment or at least to keep in control the diseased state to reduce complications. She should be healthy before conceiving a child.
4. Health status of the husband is also important as it may affect the quantity and quality of the sperm produced. Both ova and sperm are required to be healthy to produce healthy zygote and its implantation in the uterus.
5. It is important to examine the couple's blood group to screen for any blood group incompatibilities which need special care for the baby in the womb and during delivery.
6. Nutrition at the time of conception is also important. Poor nutrition status of the mother affects the pre-natal, peri-natal health and fetal growth.[25] The diet should be a balanced diet rich in vitamins and minerals. In this phase the energy requirements do not increase above normal but adequate amount of minerals and vitamins are required.

   In our community most of the females have nutritional anaemia. If mother has deficiency of iron and folic acid then the implantation of zygote is affected. Folic acid is also required for healthy growth of the embryo. It is required for formation of organs particularly brain and spinal cord. It is established in research that folic acid deficiency in mother can lead to a few congenital defects and lower I.Q. levels of the child.[26] The mother should eat diet rich in folic acid like green leafy vegetables. If she can afford, one folic acid tablet (500 μg) can be consumed daily at the time couple decides to conceive uptill 3 months of pregnancy.[27] Iron supplements should be avoided in the initial 3 months of conception.
7. The husband and wife both should avoid smoking and drinking alcohol during this phase. It affects the integrity of the sperm and ova produced and it also affects the implantation of the zygote in the mother's uterus. The mother should not smoke

at all during complete pregnancy and the father should also not smoke when the wife is around as passive smoking may also effect the growth of the fetus.

8. The healthy psychological state of the couple also contributes to healthy and efficient conception.
9. The mother should get her pregnancy status checked immediately after she notices a missed period, get registered and seek adequate health advice from the health centre.
10. The mother should get at least one ultrasound done in the 3rd month to rule out any congenital malformation in the fetus. In case any malformation is seen then the foetus can be aborted without many complications during early pregnancy period.
11. If the couple do not conceive within one year after trying, then their might be some other medical cause in either of the spouse. They both should consult an infertility specialist.

The care of the mother and child begins from the very decision for conceiving and before the time of conception. The husband and wife have to realize their collective responsibility in bearing a healthy fetus and give birth to a healthy child.

References

1. Summary of key findings from NFHS-3 2005-2006, India. Available at: http://www.nfhsindia.org/pdf/DL, pdf. Accessed on April 14, 2007.
2. Alaudin M and Maclaren L. Reaching newly wed and married adolescent. *In Focus: Focus on young adults* 1999 July;1-8.
3. WHO and UNFPA, *Married adolescent: No place for safety*, pp. 67-72, Geneva: WHO; Santhya, 2006.
4. George, A. Newly married adolescent women: Experiences from case studies in urban India. In S.Bott et al., eds, *Towards Adulthood: Exploring the Sexual and Reproductive Health of Adolescents in South Asia,* pp. 67-72, Geneva: WHO; Santhya, 2003.
5. Reproductive Health Services for Young, Engaged and Newly Married Couples. CATALYST Consortium/TAHSEEN Project funded by USAID. Available at: http://www.pathfind.org/site/Doc Server? docID=2424. Accessed on August 07, 2008.
6. Jejeebhoy, S. and K.G. Santhya. 2003. Forced sex within marriage among young women: Evidence from South Asia, presentation from

Non-consensual Sexual Experiences of Young People in Developing Countries: A Consultative Meeting, New Delhi, India, September 22-25, 2003.

7. Guyton AC, Hall JE. *Text book of Medical Physiology. ed 9th*, Prism books (Pvt.) Ltd. Bangalore 1996.
8. Zabin L, Kiragu K. The Health Consequences of Adolescent Sexual and Fertility Behaviour in Sub-Saharan Africa. *Studies in Family Planning* 1998;29(2):210-32.
9. Kanchnna V, Ojha J, Ghalot D. Significance of age in Primipara. *J Obstet Gynecol India* 1979;29:1191-5.
10. Gupta N, Mirchandani JJ. Optimum age of primigravida. *J Obstet Gynnecol India* 1978;28:767-72.
11. Community control of hereditary anemia: memorandum from a WHO meeting. *Bulletin of the World Health Organization*, 1983, 61(1):63-80.
12. Tomlinson R. China aims to improve health of newborn by law.*BMJ*. 1994 Nov 19;309(6965):1319.
13. WHO, Defining sexual health: report of a technical consultation on sexual health, 28–31 January 2002, Geneva Available at: http://www.who.int/reproductive-health/publications/sexualhealth/defining_sh.pdf. Accessed on August 07, 2008.
14. Singh S, Chaturvedi S, Kannan A.T. *Impact of a specially designed preventive intervention on some reproductive health parameters of newly married women: A prospective study.* Department of Community Medicine, University College of Medical Sciences, New Delhi; 2007. Unpublished.
15. Ibid.; and WHO, *Young People and Sexually Transmitted Diseases,* Fact Sheet, Geneva: WHO; 1997, No. 186.
16. World Health Organization (WHO), *Global Prevalence and Incidence of Selected Curable Sexually Transmitted Infections: Overview and Estimates*, Geneva: WHO; 2001.
17. WHO, *Syndromic Case Management of Sexually Transmitted Diseases*. Manila: WHO; 1997.
18. World Bank, *Improving Women's Health in India,* Washington, DC: World Bank, 1996.
19. Jejeebhoy S, Adolescent sexual and reproductive behavior: a review of the evidence from India, *Social Science & Medicine* 1998;46(10):1275–1290.

20. Devi R and Gupta SS, Awareness and health seeking behaviour of rural adolescent school girls on menstrual and reproductive health problems, *Indian Journal of Medical Science* 1999;53(10):439–443.
21. Sharan M and Valente T.W. Spousal Communication and Family Planning Adoption: Effects of a Radio Drama Serial in Nepal. *International Family Planning Perspectives* 2002 March; 28(1).
22. Kamal N, Inter-spousal communication on family planning as a determinant of the use of modern contraception in Bangladesh, *Journal of Family Welfare*, 1999, 45(1):31-43.
23. WHO, Department of Reproductive Health and Research; Family and Community Health. *Selected practice recommendations for contraceptive use*, ed 2nd. Geneva: WHO; 2004.
24. Ebrahim SH, Lo SS, Zhuo J, Han JY, Delvoye P, Zhu L. Models of preconception care implementation in selected countries. *Matern Child Health J*. 2006 Sep;10(5 Suppl):S37-42.
25. Baveja R, Agarwal R, Pal A, Mukherjee K, Mishra R. Maternal nutrition assessment and fetal outcome. *J Obstet Gynecol India* 1993;43:469-72.
26. Bundage SC. Preconception health care. *Am Fam Physician* 2002 Jun 15;65:2507-14.
27. Berry RJ, Li Z, Erickson JD. Li S, Moore CA, Wang H, et al. Prevention of neural tube defects with folic acid in China. *N Engl J Med* 1999; 341: 1485-1490.

32

PILES – non Medicinal Management

Ravinder Kumar and AJ Singh

Common man call them piles, the aristocracy call them hemorrhoids. Believe it or not, about 10 million people in the world are affected by troublesome piles every year. Prevalence of piles is reported to be 40% in India and as high as 60% in western world. Women are suffering from piles more than man.

What are Piles

Piles are akin to, but not the same as, varicose veins and piles only occur in the anal region, enlarged, dilated veins of the hemorrhoid plexuses (hemorrhoid plexuses being the network of blood vessels of the lower rectum and anal canal, to be medically precise).

The veins in this area of human body are quite flexible and stretchable to coexist with the bowel expanding and contracting. This is why piles can only occur in this area of the body - no other veins in the body can stretch as much and become so huge when pressurised with blood.

The piles, as such, develops when one of the weakened veins expands under pressure - such as when straining on the toilet.

Once expanded and if unable to return to normal size, it is then called piles.

Types of Piles

If the engorged vein is outside the anus, but really close to it, it is described as an external hemorrhoid *or piles*. Specifically, external hemorrhoids have three main symptoms: They are seen as little bleeding areas that occur under the skin near the anus, which can be felt as hard lumps. They also do not show through the opening, but develop more on the rim, just outside and, because external hemorrhoids develop in the often darkened area of skin near the opening, they are often brownish in color.

If the engorged vein is inside, it is referred to as an *internal hemorrhoid or piles* although they may bleed; they are seldom painful unless infected.

If the engorged vein is internal, but hangs outside where you can see it or feel it, it is referred to as a hemorrhoid prolapse or a *prolapsed hemorrhoid* and, they are generally reddish in color.

Aetiology of Piles

Heredity is a definitely a predisposing factor, such as congenital weakness of the vein walls. Piles are rare in quadrupeds because of their horizontal orientation in which the venous blood is flows in the body parallel to the earth. But in man, because of his vertical orientation the weight of the column of blood produces a high venous pressure in the lower rectum. So, man is more prone to get piles.

Straining accompanying the constipation or that induced by the overpurgation is also a potent cause of the piles. Straining at micturition because of urethral strictures or enlarged prostate or doing coughing or lifting the heavy objects are the other equally important causes of the piles. Diarrhoea can also aggravate the latent piles. Pregnancy also result the piles, due to compression of the veins by the uterus and effect of the hormones on the smooth muscle in the walls of the veins.

Sypmtoms of Piles

When the piles initially show themselves, the common reaction is one of shock, fear and concern. Patient feels pain, itch and burn like nothing one ever experienced before. For some it's the shock of seeing lots of blood suddenly coming out or severe excruciating pain from a thrombosed piles. Fortunately, all the types of piles really are swollen blood vessels, which for most people, are easily cured or relieved. Self diagnosis of piles is difficult. A lay person may confuse piles with warts, abscess, anal fissure, anal prolapse, cancer or other conditions.

1. The common appearances of real piles

The most obvious symptom of piles is that they are often felt and seen (for example, by using a mirror) as a tiny lump of grapes arising from the anus. The size, shape and number of piles vary from one person to another. A pile can be larger than a grape, even walnut size, but typically they are the size of a pea. Piles can look like flattened grapes, some look like full grapes, while others may look wrinkly. Piles may come out of the anus, that is protrude, other times the piles remain inside the anus out of view, while some piles develop on the skin outside of the anus. Reddish pink piles are normally prolapsed internal hemorrhoids. Purple blue or dark reddish piles are normally thrombosed hemorrhoids. Brown piles are often external hemorrhoids.

2. More common signs and symptoms of piles

A very annoying symptom of piles is that they can cause one's bottom to become itchy, particularly round the anal opening. Piles can also cause a burning sensation, pain and or discomfort around the anal opening. Soiling of underwear can be a common symptom with piles as well. This piles symptom can cause the other symptoms of itching and burning - akin to nappy rash. Piles can also cause a feeling of incomplete evacuation of the bowel - one doesn't feel like having emptied his bowels even after doing so.

Some symptoms of piles are used as the basis of classifying piles into grades:

Grade 1 hemorrhoids do not prolapse, may bleed. Grade 2 hemorrhoids prolapse - pop out - when straining, but the hemorrhoids go back in of their own accord; they may bleed. Grade 3 hemorrhoids pop out when straining, tend to bleed more and have to be gently pushed back in. Grade 4 hemorrhoids are showing all the time and bleed much more.

MANAGEMENT OF PILES WITHOUT MEDICINES AT HOME

All the cases of piles necessarily not require expensive medical treatment. There are many popular home remedies for this ailment

1. Diet and Fibre : Fiber and diet is likely the most important point to develop a piles treatment at the home. The high fiber diet is suitable for constipation, piles and other conditions

The high fiber diet: Why a high fiber diet? Constipation causes piles by causing pressure on the hemorrhoidal area and hard stools are more likely to cause piles to bleed by scratching them. Every human being needs between twenty to thirty grams of fiber per day in their diet. Fiber is not broken down by the gastrointestinal system, but is rather passed through it serving as regulator and scrubber at the same time. 30 grams of fiber is what is desirable in a high fiber diet. The best way to get enough fiber is to consume whole grains, fresh fruits and vegetables, and the ever popular beans. Getting fiber through your diet is the best option because these foods carry vital nutrients and trace minerals as well as constipation-banishing fiber.

Common foods for a high fiber diet: Most fruits and vegetables have 2 to 3 grams fiber per 100 gms and therefore good for a high fiber diet. Nuts and seeds have around 3 gms fiber per 30 gm serving.

Fruits: Apple - 1x200g large with skin, but cored - 6.0 gms fiber, Guava - 1 x 120 gm medium 6.5 gms fiber, Orange - 1x300g large - 5.5 gms, Peach - 1x225g large - 4 gms, Pear - 1x200gms large - 6 gms

Salads: Bean salad - 1/2 cup - 5 gms

Vegetables: Peas / snow peas - 100 gm - 4.5 gm

Lentils and beans: Have about 5 grams of fiber per 100 grams cooked.

Fibers and Water: If a high fiber diet is included in your constipation and piles diet, then water becomes very important to it. In addition to getting enough fiber, you'll want to drink at least eight decent-sized glasses of water per day. Taking a high fiber diet without getting enough water is about as sensible as eating glue, and that's exactly what it'll feel like in your stomach. Fiber absorbs excess water, which produces the sort of firm, easy to pass stools that will convince your constipation and haemorrhoids to go away.

2. Using the Toilet : Yes, going the correct way on a toilet is also vital to most piles home remedy plans, as will be shown below:

Staying on the toilet for more than five minutes at a time may also aggravate or worsen your piles. Limit your time on the toilet, because if you don't go within a few minutes, it's better to wait till later than let your hemorrhoids hang there and get worse. If it's a western type of latrines, get a footstool to put your feet up on while sitting, whether on the toilet or anywhere else. **Using a squatting toilet (Indian Type) may also help**, as a squatting position does not rob you of the support of any of your pelvic muscles, while a sitting toilet does.

Thus Western toilets predispose you to piles, while use of Indian type latrine prevents development of piles.

*3. Physical activities: don't just sit or stand :*Take several short walks a day, as too much sitting or just plain standing can upset piles. So be sure to include this in your piles home remedy plan, if you sit or stand for long stretches at a time.

4. Sleep with legs raised if possible : As part of your basic piles home remedy plan, finding a way to sleep overnight with your legs elevated (putting a pillow below legs) can do wonders for relieving the blood pressure on hemorrhoidal veins.

5. Suitable ointments and creams : The most common and probably most effective ingredient is a lubricant and a moisturizer. Cocoa butter, petroleum jelly, and glycerin compounds are the most popular and are easily available at home. Piles tend to become sore from being chaffed when outside the anal opening, so a little bit of cream soothes the piles quite well and stops them being chaffed further.

6. Sitz baths : are one very popular piles home remedy. Sitz baths help to alleviate piles symptoms such as inflammation, itching and swelling. This is one of the most popular home remedies for piles. For immediate relief from either internal or external hemorrhoids, many people find warm, plain water baths to be helpful. Draw 2 to 3 inches (5 to 8 cm) of water that is as warm or hot as you can stand it, and sit in it for twenty minutes three times per day. Right after the bath, sitting on a towel-wrapped ice pack is often both beneficial and soothing. The alternating of heat and cold gets the blood in the area moving again, which is all to the good when it comes to piles.

7. *Appropriate physical care of piles*: is another good home remedy for pain relief and easing discomfort. Another good practice with piles is, if needed, to use mild soap and water to cleanse the area after using the toilet paper or to use a soft cloth with soap and water is much easier on the piles than repeated wiping with toilet paper.

8. *Appropriate toilet paper*: (for those who use the toilet paper) is a simple home remedy. Also, with external or protruding piles, a soft toilet paper can be worth its weight in gold for preventing and reducing pile pain. Cheap, hard toilet paper is likely to upset pile pretty badly, particularly if you have to keep wiping the piles to get reasonably clean. Fluids emitted by the intestinal tract in the normal daily course of doing it's job, which is to break down food, can often be irritating to tender piles, so clean gently and well with cool water and plain, hypoallergenic soap at least once per day. Patting the area clean after bowel movements with pads soaked in aloe vera, or apple vinegar is good both for cleaning and to dry and soothe the area as an alternative to wiping with toilet paper.

9. *Reinsertion* is a very effective home remedy for prolapsed piles. One can also try to gently push the piles back into the anus - if that is where they are coming from - but be careful not to damage them. Once the piles are pushed back in, the pain should subside very quickly.

10. *The Haemorrhoid cushion* is a home remedy for piles relief that has been practised for many years. Some piles sufferers find relief from using a hemorrhoid cushion. A piles cushion is normally an inflatable rubber ring, similar to the inflatable rings that kids wear at the pool or beach. You sit on it, rather than wear

it. The piles cushion works essentially by removing or minimizing contact pressure between the sitting surface and the piles, as well as by possibly relieving the pressure of the backside cheeks on any prolapsed piles. A soft cushion or pillow may also help relieve the piles symptoms when sitting.

11. The use of ice can help to reduce swelling and pain of piles. We all know that ice packs help reduce swelling, One can either shape a piece of ice into a suppository shape - akin to a rifle bullet, but not as long and with rounded ends, or you can let some ice cubes melt to they are about the same sort of shape. One should make sure the ice is wet and slippery and not sticky to the skin. Insert it like a normal suppository.

12. Avoiding tight fitting undergarments, should be included as an easy piles home remedy. Tight fitting clothing irritates piles because it can restrict blood flow to the area and puts further inflaming pressure on the piles in question. Tight clothing and underwear can also be both irritating to the area and contributes to low muscle tone, which is part of the underlying issue that leads to piles. In addition, some people are sufficiently sensitive to the synthetic materials that underwear can be made of as to make already existing hemorrhoids worse.

13. Exercise and Yoga should be part of any piles home remedy plan. There are a few mechanical tricks that can be used to treat and banish piles as well. The first and simplest is to get the blood moving, which is accomplished by increased activity. If you have a job that requires long periods of sitting or standing, take a break and a brisk walk for five minutes every two hours or so. With your doctor's consent, start walking for half an hour, three times a week. Doing yoga, where you clench and release all of your pelvic muscles ten times, will help you regain and retain the muscle tone needed to support anorectal veins. *Matsya Aasan, Srisha Asan, Surya Namaskara, Tada Asana and Sarvanga Asana* are the most useful *yoga asanas* for control of piles.

References

1. J.E.L. Sales, M.Chir, "Anus and Rectum" Outpatient Surgery, W.B. Sounders Company. 1980; 2nd edition:1122.

2. Ira j. Kodner, Robert D.Fry, James W. Fleshmina, "Colon Rectum and Anus" Schwartz's Principles of Surgery, Vol. 2.1999;7th edition:1295-1296.
3. A.J. Harding, H. David Ritchie. "The Anal canal and Rectum" Bailey and Love's A short Practice of Surgery, ELBS London,1985; 19th edition:1041.
4. W. Hamish Thomsons. "Hemmorroids or Piles" Oxford textbook of surgery, Oxford University Press, NewYork 2000; 2nd edition:1553.
5. http://www.hemorrhoidshemroids.com/index.html accessed on 12/07/008.
6. Roger D.Dazios, "Disorders of the Anal Canal" Sabistons The Textbook of Surgery. W.B.Sounders Company1997;15 th edition:1036.
7. Jose R.Cintra, Marc A. Singer, "Hemmorroids" Current surgical therapy. Mosby Inc.St. Louis.2001;7thedition:273-274.
8. http://www.hemorrhoidshemroids.com/hemroids-hemorrhoids-home-remedy.html accessed on 12/07/08.
9. http://www.yogawiz.com/askquestion/697/treatment-for-piles-how-to-cure-piles-through-yoga.html accessed on 15/07/08.

33

Self Care in Pregnancy

Avinash Rana, Vanita Suri, Indarjit Walia and AJ Singh

INTRODUCTION

With the rapid pace of industrialization and urbanization in today's society, the joint family system has broken down. Earlier, elderly women in joint families used to guide/tell pregnant women about maternity/child care. In every family, there used to be many married women living together who shared their experiences and helped each other regarding various aspects of motherhood/ maternity. With the breakdown of joint family system, there is usually no one in the family to guide the women on these issues.

Such problems are particularly faced by the women who become pregnant for the first time. It has been reported that primigravida women often lack knowledge on various aspects of pregnancy, labor, postpartum care and neonatal care e.g. diet, rest, precautions, appropriate postures while working during pregnancy, recognition of true labor pains, diet and hydration during labor etc. Now, all this has been medicalized. The traditional birth attendants who used to take care of maternity related issues in families are also vanishing. The role of the family members & TBA has been taken over by the hospital set up. Nurses and doctors are now expected to tell primigravida women about maternity care which was considered earlier an internal family matter. However, most of the time of nurses / obstetricians is spent in clinical care.

Consequently, they have little time to attend to routine day to day advisory needs of pregnant women. The situation is particularly more critical in India where because of its population size hospital is overcrowded. Moreover, in government health care set up in India, female doctors are scarce and are overworked; they are not able to devote adequate time to individual pregnant women. Consequently, in this set up, preparedness of most primigravida for safe motherhood leaves much to be desired.[1,2]

So, evidently, general public and the clients of maternal health care services need to be educated about some basics aspects of pregnancy care and related issues. For such empowerment of the people, health education strategies have been devised to propagate self care.

The concept of self-care was evolved to empower patients to enable them to take care of their routine lives so that they are not dependent on doctor/nurses. Implementation of this concept requires that the health care professionals impart skills of self care to the women. Nurses and midwives have an important role in this endeavor. Dissemination of health related information to the family and community has been projected as one of the primary functions of the nurses / midwives in promoting the health of antenatal women and helping them to attain their optimum state of well being.[3-6].

Health education during pregnancy seeks to enable the pregnant women to actively participate in their own antenatal care with or without the help of nurse or obstetrician. In fact, for primigravida her pregnancy is fraught with many uncertainties. For her the course of pregnancy is an unknown path .There are so many physiological changes during pregnancy and so many likely complications that may occur during antenatal period. However, do's & don'ts during labor are not known to many women, particularly the first timers. . Many women are not aware of the guidelines pertaining to these issues. This makes them apprehensive about the course and outcome of the pregnancy. Their anxiety level is also high. Proper knowledge about these things will prepare the women adequately for labor. There are many things women may be taught so that it improves the outcome. e.g. what to eat , what to wear, how to prepare for labor , how to recognize the onset of, labor, what to do when one has cramps , what test to get done etc [7,8].

Similar to the lack of awareness of primigravida about what to do during nine months of pregnancy, there are many more serious issues as to when it comes to the actual delivery itself i.e. how to go about delivering the baby. Primigravida enter the labor room with an unprepared yet apprehensive frame of mind. Labor support has several components, including physical comfort, emotional support, patient teaching or giving information, and advocacy. Labor support is considered to be an important part of intrapartum nurses role, yet most studies have suggested that only a minimal nursing time is spent for providing supportive care. This is because mostly doctor and nurses are too busy to explain the women about what should they do to facilitate labor. Similarly women, particularly primigravida , do not know what to do just after the delivery . There are many things beyond the immediate medical concern that are not known to women but are crucial for their as well as their babies welfare. These aspects need to be taught to women well in advance.[9-11]

Childbirth educators can have a significant impact on safe care for mothers and babies during labor and birth. Pregnant women and their families need accurate, scientific information to advocate for themselves and their care in full partnership with nurses, nurse midwives, and physicians. In addition to focusing on what to expect during labor and how to handle contraction pain and discomfort, pregnant women are often concerned about their ability to push their baby out when the time comes. They may hear from friends and family of long, exhausting hours of pushing while, in contrast, they observe television portrayals of women who usually give birth after only one or two pushes. Information presented in childbirth preparation classes provides a foundation for expectations of how care will be provided and what women need to know to safely complete the last part of labor before birth.

Often, women receive conflicting advice regarding maternity care from their friends, relatives or neighbors. Many of them are confused about what to believe, especially primigravida mothers, who are often shy and reluctant to ask questions. Following guidelines (which have been successfully tested by the authors as a part of PhD thesis work involving a randomized controlled trial) attempt to educate the women about self care for minor problems during pregnancy and labor. Instructions are also given regarding self care of mother and the child after delivery.

Minor Disorders in Pregnancy

1. BACKACHE

- As your baby grows your posture changes.
  This puts extra stress on your back and thighs.
- Hormones of pregnancy relax your joints.
- As breasts gain in size and weight, the result is a stooped posture.
  Above 3 changes are the possible causes of backache.

WHAT YOU CAN DO	DON'T
· Wear low-heeled shoes/slippers with equal level of sole.	Lift heavy weight e.g. bucket full of water
· Do abdominal wall exercises (blow out exhale and pull in your abdominal wall for the count of 5).	Do heavy exercises
· Practice pelvic tilt exercises	
· Do shoulder circles forwards and backwards.	
· Stand with your back against a wall. Place a hand in the small of your back then drop your hand.	
· Bend your knees when lifting, (basket/bucket etc)	Lift weight without bending knee
· Hold objects as close to your body as possible when you want to lift it.	Hold objects away from your body while lifting
· When standing for long periods rest one foot on a stool	Stand for long periods
· Regularly rotate your feet in small circles	Rotate your feet too fast
· Use the strength of your legs when getting up.	

CORRECT POSTURES

In most of the cases problem of backache is due to wrong posture. It can be prevented if correct posture is maintained.

CORRECT POSTURE (A)

A. STANDING (FIG. 3)

DO'S	DON'TS
· Stand comfortably	Stand on slippery floor
· Keep your feet straight on forward the floor	Bend your shoulders and backward
· Keep your arms straight by the side of the body	Bend your arms
· Keep your neck and head straight	Bend your neck and head forward

CORRECT POSTURE (B)

B. Sit comfortably on the floor, chair/sofa, bed, *peedhi / chownki*

FLOOR (Fig. 1)

DO'S

- Sit on clean floor
- Keep your buttocks touching the floor
- Keep your legs straight flexed on the floor
- Sit in a butterfly position (Fig. 4)

DON'TS

- Sit on slippery floor
- Keep your buttocks above the floor level

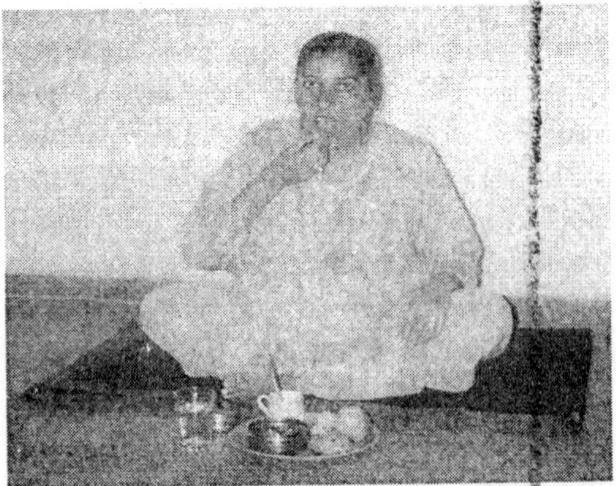

Fig. 1

CHAIR/SOFA

DO'S (Fig. 2)

- Sit comfortable on the Chair /sofa
- Support the back against the back of the chair/sofa
- Keep feet on the floor or on the *peedhi* / *chownki*

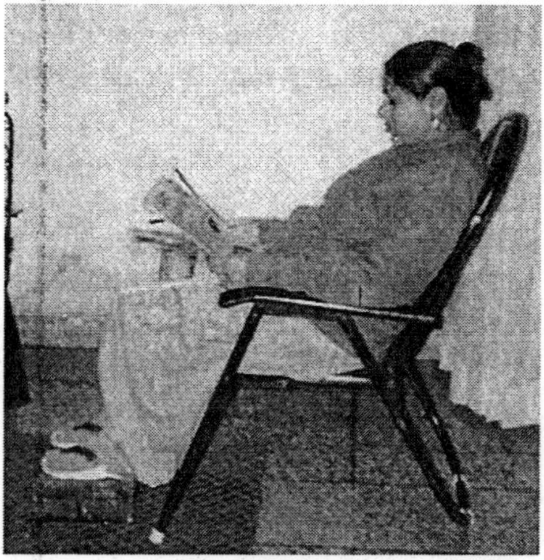

Fig. 2

DON'TS (Fig. 3)

- Sit on too small a chair
- Sit on broken chair/sofa
- Let feet hang in the air
- Leave a gap between your back and the back of chair/sofa

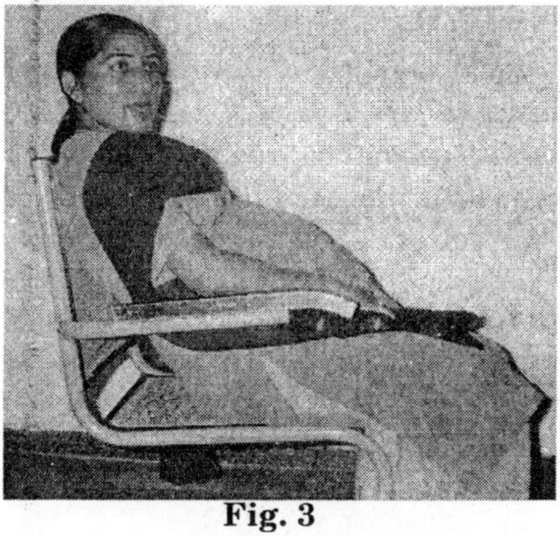

Fig. 3

CHOWNKI / PEEDHI

DO'S	DON'TS
· Sit on *peedhi / chownki* as you like	Sit on very small *peedhi / chownki*
· Keep your buttocks on it	
· Keep your feet touching the floor	Use broken *peedhi / chownki*

CORRECT POSTURE (C)
LYING DOWN (Fig. 4)

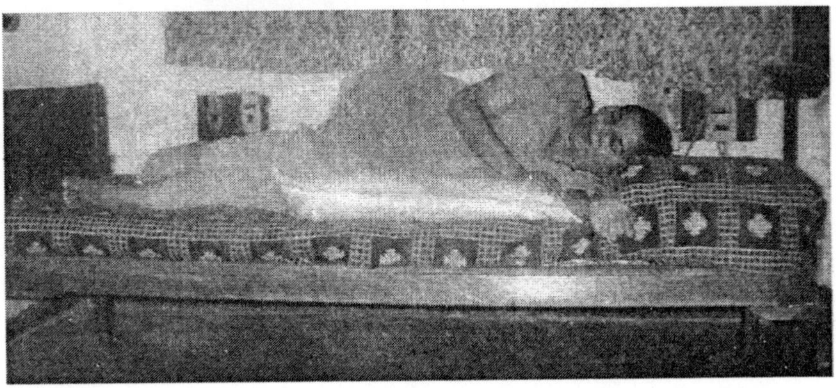

Fig. 4

DO'S	DON'TS
· Rest in hard bed with firm mattress	Lie down in too loose bed *navar / cane* bed
· Lie down in lateral (either posture position)	Lie down in straight
· Keep one / two pillows under head / knee	Keep too many pillows under the head\knee

GETTING UP FROM BED (FIG. 5)

DO'S	DON'TS
· Get up slowly	Get up very fast
· Change positions slowly	Change positions too fast
· Roll over to your side. Use your arms to bring your body to a sitting position. Bring your legs down/feet should touch the floor	Do a "sit up"

· Sit for 2-3 minutes on the bed and then get up from the bed	Start walking immediately when you get down from bed

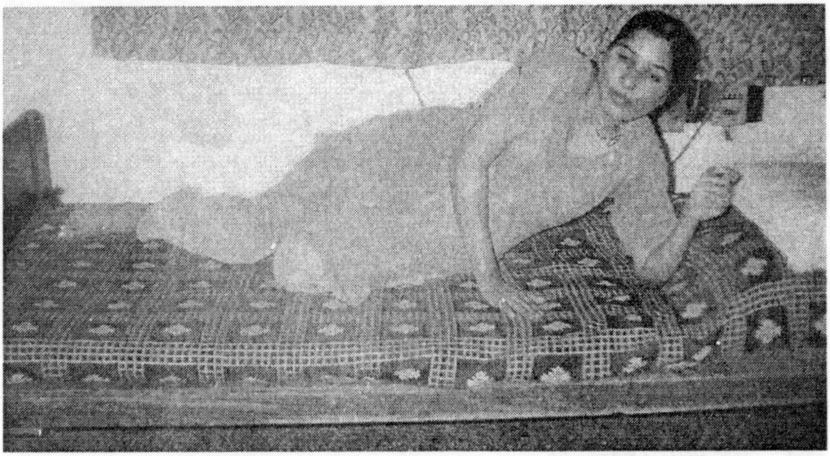

Fig. 5

2. **CRAMPS IN YOUR LEGS**

Cause:

- Increased pressure on the nerves in your abdomen by the growing baby.
- Extra strain on your legs due to standing for long duration

Symptoms:

- Sudden pain in the calf muscles (lower leg)
- Difficulty in walking

DO'S	DON'T
· Take rest in between where long standing required	Stand for long time
· Take a pint of milk (three glasses) in a day	Forget to take milk.

HOW TO RELIEVE CRAMPS

(a) **With the help of another person (Fig. 6)**

During cramps another person forces the foot upwards towards the abdomen with one hand on the sole of the feet below the toes, while the woman keeps legs straight by putting pressure on the hand of that person

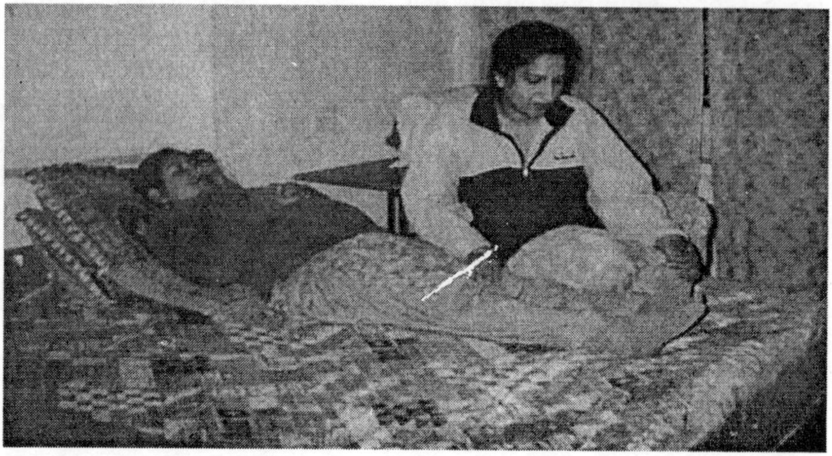

Fig. 6

(b) By self (Fig. 7)

· Gently push your feet against a firm surface

· Gently stretch your leg against wall/chair

* keep your hands on the wall /chair

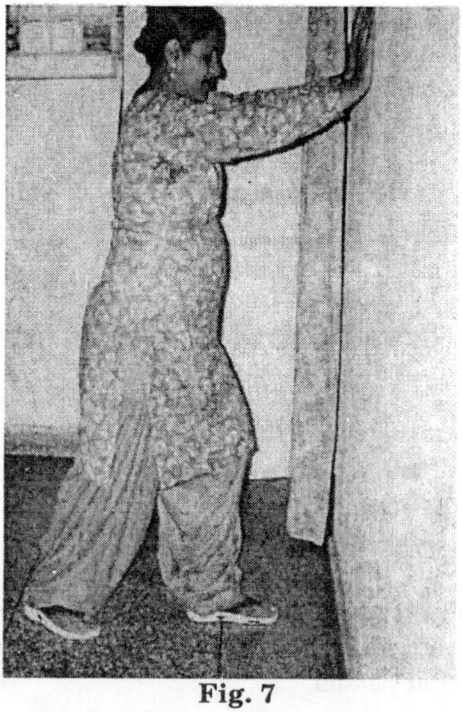

Fig. 7

- put pressure against the wall
- stretch your legs
- keep your feet on the floor
- Put your feet up several times during the day

3. VARICOSE VEINS

- The flow of blood from the peripheral parts of the body to heart is slowed because of pressure exerted by your growing baby on the veins.
- The increased fluid in your blood stream and slowed blood flow cause swollen veins.

SYMPTOMS

Pain and tiredness in the lower extremities

- Feeling of heaviness in varicosities in the vulva and perineum
- Redness heat and tenderness at the site.

DO'S	DON'TS
· Regular walk	cross your legs/feet while sitting
· Put your feet up several times for a day on a stool / *peedhi*	Stand / sit in one position long period
· Elevate your legs with hips when you sit	
· During long sitting / standing periods(unavoidable reason) walk frequently to promote venous return to the heart	
· Do foot exercises (As given in self care) (Fig. 13)	Do foot exercises if injury on the ankle.

STEPS (FOOT EXERCISES)

DO'S	DON'TS
(A)	
· Dorsiflex the feet (pull upwards)	Do dorsiflex the foot too forcefully
· Hold above position for 3 seconds then release	
· Repeat above exercise for 8-10 times each day	

(B)

· Lie down with your legs elevated one pillow lying down under one hip elevated(to avoid compression of the veins)	Keep too many pillows while on pillows and place

4. VARICOSITIES OF VULVA AND ANUS

· Aches and sense of heaviness on the vulva and perineum

DO'S	DON'TS
· Take lots of water	Forget to take fluids
· Apply perineal pad for support and anus	Leave the varicosities of vulva without support
· Lie down in Sim's position i.e. keep one pillow under the head. Lie down in left side, straighten the left leg and place the left arm at the back side slightly in flexed position. Flex and place your right arm on the head pillow and right leg on the other pillow.	Lie down in straight position

5. FAINTING SPELLS

· Feeling of dizziness for few seconds.

DO'S	DON'TS
· Lie on your left side	Lie down supine or straight on your back
· Sit down immediately and lower your head between the legs, when you feel uneasy / dizzy.	Start walking immediately
· Take sweet/sugar immediately	Be in hurry
· Take glucose water	Take extra sweet/sugar if
· Get blood pressure checked up	you have diabetes

PREVENTION

- Arise slowly from resting position
- Change positions slowly
- Avoid prolonged standing in warm/stuffy environment
- Make sure you are eating and drinking enough at regular times

- Always keep some toffees in your pocket/purse
- Wear loose clothes

6. HEART BURN

- Burning and irritation in the food pipe which goes upwards leaving bad taste in the mouth.

CAUSE

- Due to displacements of the stomach by enlarging uterus.

DO'S	DON'TS
· Eat small and frequent meals	Take those food that make you feel uncomfortable.
· Walk for 10-15 minutes in the room after each meal	Lie down 2 hours after a meal
· Sleep with your head raised on a pillow	Take medicine unless suggested by doctor
	Take fried / fatty food
· Take last meals at least 2 hours before bed time	

REMEDY

- Drink adequate amount of fluids each day.
- Take frequent sips of milk / water
- Take 10 ml chilled milk without sugar
- Take one table spoon antacid (Gel) before meal.

7. CONSTIPATION

- Difficult to pass hard stool.

CAUSES:

- As your baby grows, it puts more pressure on your bowel obstructing it.

DO'S	DON'TS
· Drink 6-8 glasses of fluids every day	Forget to take water / fluids
· Take a glass of warm water in the morning before tea/breakfast	Take any laxatives (Anticonstipation) medicine unless advised by doctor

· Add more fruits and vegetables (spinach, cabbage, *sag* etc) in your meal	Take *maida* made stuff such as pizza, bread etc.
· Exercise regularly 3 to 4 times a week	
· Go for morning and evening walk	

8. PILES

- Pressure on blood vessels in your rectum can cause a slowing of the blood flow and swelling of the veins.
- It may cause burning, itching and sometimes bleeding

DO'S	DON'TS
· Lie on your side while resting	
· Do pelvic floor exercises.	Sit / stand too long
· Reduce the swelling by raising your hips and legs several times a day	
· Apply ice / cold packs and cream	Do fomentation hemorrhoid
· Take advice if you have severe pain	
· Go to doctor if piles persists	Take any medicine without doctor's advice
· Avoid constipation	

9. SWELLING (FEET, HANDS, ANKLES)

- Some swelling on your feet below the ankle is normal but if it is increasing; involves your hands and face, consult a doctor.

CAUSE

- Extra fluid in your body
- Pressure on blood vessels in your pelvis by your growing baby

DO'S	DON'TS
· Get blood pressure checked frequently	
· Put your feet up as often as possible	Stand/walk for long periods

· Go to doctor if finger ring is tight	
· Rest and sleep on your left side	Stay in one position for long periods
· Use normal amount of salt and avoid potato-chips, soft drinks preserved meats and pickles	Add extra salt in diet
· Exercise regularly.	
· Wear support stockings. Put them on before you get out of bed in the morning	Reduce your fluids
· Sudden excessive swelling may be a sign of HIGH BLOOD PRESSURE, see your doctor immediately	Wear tight clothes rings, and shoes.

10. SLEEPLESSNESS OR INSOMNIA

DO'S	DON'TS
· Daily walk in the evening	Do exhausting walk in the evening
· Take a glass of warm milk at bed time	Take rest less than 2 hours
· Read story book	Read books till late night
· Wear loose clothes at night	Wear tight clothes
· Take frequent rest in between before you become overtired	Use more than two pillows
· Use extra pillow for comfort when you lie on your side. Place one small pillow between your knees and one behind your back (Fig. ___).	Under your head
· During the day take short breaks with your feet up.	
· Do light Exercise regularly	Forget to do regular exercise.
· Reduce caffeine intake	Take too much caffeine.

11. CRAVINGS (PICA)

- When you crave for certain foods or unnatural substances such as clay (*mitti*), coal, *rajasthani mitti, pickles* etc

CAUSES

- Due to changes in the body

DO'S	DON'TS
· Eat well balanced diet	Eat unnatural substances too much
· Take advice from doctor / nurse if you consume too much unnatural substances	Feel shy to ask the doctor/ nurse if you are crave for unnatural substances

12. SKIN CHANGES

- Dark discoloration on face, breasts, abdomen and thighs.

CAUSES

- Due to stretching of the skin during pregnancy

DO'S	DON'T'S
· Wear loose clothes	Scratch on the abdomen
· Apply cold cream	Neglect if itching present along with yellow discoloration of the skin (it may be due to jaundice or if more at night time may be scabies).

13. FREQUENT PASSING OF URINE

- As your baby is pressing on your bladder

DO'S	DONT'S
· Drink 6-8 glasses of fluid in a day.	Reduce the amount of fluids that you drink
· Do pelvic floor exercises (pull up and tighten the pelvic floor muscles as if you are stopping the flow of urine)	Take too much caffeine
· Repeat this exercise 5 to 10 times, several time a day	Practice the exercise while passing urine

· Wash your perineal area with soap water and dry it after voiding.	Forget to wash your perineal area
· Wear clean underwear.	
· Consult doctor, if pain, burning pain or hematuria occur	Delay to consult doctor, if burning or hematuria occurs.

DANGER SIGNALS IN PREGNANCY AND THEIR MANAGEMENT

THINGS TO BE KEPT IN MIND WHEN YOU ARE SHIFTING TO HOSPITAL BECAUSE OF EMERGENCY

- Do not Panic.
- Keep clean perineal pad (in case of bleeding / leakage per vagina).
- Always lie down on left lateral position during transportation.
- Keep some help ready (Extra hand / money).

Danger Signals in Pregnancy

- Every delivery is a risk situation
- Risk can lead to death or disease of the MOTHER & BABY
- This can be avoided or minimized by early detection of such risks and relevant remedial measures.

1. VAGINAL BLEEDING BEFORE THE BIRTH OF THE BABY

- Any type of bleeding per vagina before the birth of the baby can be dangerous for the mother / baby. It may be with / without pains. **If you have such bleeding, rush to the hospital immediately** (or consult a doctor).

What to do (till you reach hospital)

- Keep clean perineal pad
- Lie down in left lateral position
- Save all the perineal pads and show to the doctor when you reach hospital (to estimate loss of blood)
- Tell the doctor whether bleeding p/v before or started after onset of labour pains

· Move to the hospital as early as possible	Do not eat or drink any thing except water
· Avoid internal examination by dai or others	

2. PREMATURE RUPTURE / BREAK OF BAG OF WATER

- In the womb baby floats in a bag of water. This bag can rupture any time anywhere during pregnancy with / without labour pains. Warm liquid may also dribble out or gush profusely with / without labour pain.

What to do

AT HOME	IN HOSPITAL
· Note the time when leakage started	Show the perineal pad to the doctor
· Keep a clean pad as you keep during menstruation	Tell the doctor what time the leakage started
Lie down on left lateral side	
· See the color of leakage whether it is like clear water, green / yellow in colour	
· If it is clear / green / yellow / blood stained in colour without delay come to the hospital immediately	Do not take anything by mouth (there may be the need of operation)
· Lie down on left lateral position during transportation	

3. GREENISH FLUID COMES OUT OF VAGINA BEFORE THE BIRTH OF THE BABY

- Normally baby do not pass stool inside the womb. But under stress the unborn baby passes stools in the womb. It indicate that there is some problem inside the womb. If transportation to the hospital is delayed the unborn baby may aspirate this greenish fluid. This can kill the baby. Immediate action has to be taken.

What to do

IN HOME	IN HOSPITAL
· Keep clean perineal pad	Show the perineal pad to the doctor
· Lie down in left lateral position	Lie down in left lateral position
· Do not take any thing by mouth (There may be need of operation)	Do not panic if operation is advised

4. ANY CHANGE IN FETAL MOVEMENTS

- Any change in fetal movements indicate fetus is at stress. Always keep record of your baby's movements.

How to count fetal movements

- Sit comfortably on the chair or bed one hour after each meal (breakfast, lunch, dinner)
- Lie down on left lateral side.
- Keep pen/pencil and a diary or paper
- Keep your hand on upper abdomen
- Feel whenever baby moves and record with pencil on the paper
- Record the fetal movements for 3 hours (till one hour after every meal – breakfast, lunch and dinner) if the count is less then 10-12 movements in three flows/less than 3 movements per hour approach the doctor.

What to do

IN HOME	IN HOSPITAL
· Keep accurate record of fetal movements with date and time. (6th month onwards)	
· Lie down on lateral side to feel fetal movement for 1 hour. Count for another hour if no movements then immediately come to the hospital	Show the fetal movements chart to the doctor.

5. PERSISTENT HEADACHE, BLURRING VISION, SUDDEN AND SEVERE VOMITING

- If you have these together, these are the signs of high blood pressure.

What to do

AT HOME	IN HOSPITAL
· Immediately lie down on left lateral side	Don't be anxious
· Immediately come to hospital with one/two family members If you have headache	Lie down in lateral side

Other family members

· Transfer her very comfortably to hospital	Don't go to toilet. Use bed pan
· If fit / convulsions occur at home/ on the way put spoon above the tongue to prevent tongue bite	Give proper history of convulsions to the doctor

6. PREMATURE LABOUR PAINS

- When labor pains start within 7th to 9th months (28 weeks to 36 weeks) it is known as premature labour.
- S/s:- Cramps (may feel like menstrual cramps/gas pain)
- low back pain and uterus becomes hard
- fluid gush or leakage of fluid from birth canal
- change/increase in vaginal discharge
- full/heavy feeling in the birth passage (vagina)

What to do at home

AT HOME	IN HOSPITAL
· Immediately rush to the hospital	
· Don't panic	Lie down in lateral position.
· Keep clean perineal pad in underwear if there is leakage or blood discharge p/v.	
· Lie down in lateral side	
· Be prepared. Baby may be too small. It will need special care/ incubator care.	

7. PROLONGED LABOUR (More than 12 hours)

- When labour pains are very strong and contractions are painful but ineffective to open the mouth of the uterus and last more than 12 hours without result.

What to do

AT HOME	IN HOSPITAL
· Take deep breath during labour pains through nose and exhale labour through the lips	Give complete history (since how long continuously pains are there)
· Lie down on lateral side	Lie down on lateral side
· Move to the hospital without any delay	
· Do not take anything by mouth	

8. PAIN IN ABDOMEN

- Never ignore pain in lower abdomen in pregnancy. It can be dangerous for your baby.

What to do

AT HOME	AT HOSPITAL
· Note the characteristic of pain – Does it start from back & comes forward.	Give complete history of abdominal pain whether it was accompanied with bleeding per vaginally
· Note if there is any bleeding per vaginally. Keep perineal pad in the undergarments	Lie down on lateral position
· Lie down on left lateral side	
· Don't take any medicine to relieve the pain.	

SELF CARE IN PREGNANCY

1. HYGIENE

- Daily hygiene is important during pregnancy because of the increase in perspiration and vaginal discharge caused by hormonal changes.

2. BATHING

- Take daily bath with soap & water.
- Sit on the stool/*chownki* while taking bath.
- Keep your feet very carefully against slipping in the bathroom.
- Always wear rough surface sole *chappal* (avoid slippery soles).
- Regular scrubbing of the bathroom floor should be done.

3. BREAST CARE

- Keep your breasts clean.
- Wash them daily with soap & water while taking bath.
- Wear well fitted/supportive bra.
- Examine for any abnormality.
- Do nipples exercises if nipples are inverted (nipples are facing inward).

Nipple Rolling (Fig. 8)

- Gently pull them between thumb and index finger.
- Hold them in this position for 1-2 minutes.
- Repeat this for 5-6 times during bath.

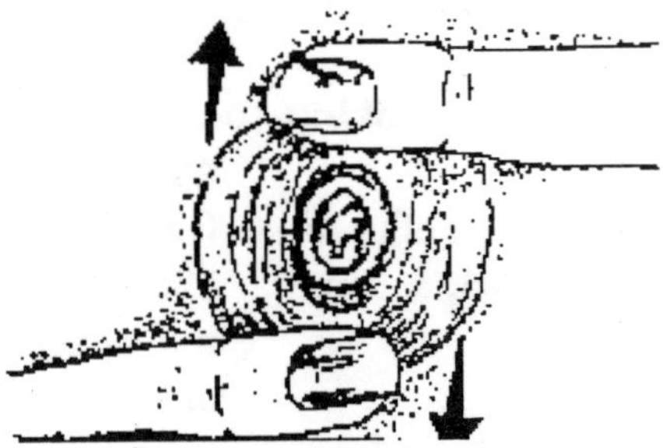

Fig. 8

Nipple-Stretching (Fig. 9)

- Place thumb/index fingers opposite each other near the edge of the dark part (Areola) of the breast.
- Press the breast and stretch outward.
- Hold them in this position for 1-2 minutes.
- Repeat this for 5-6 times during bath.

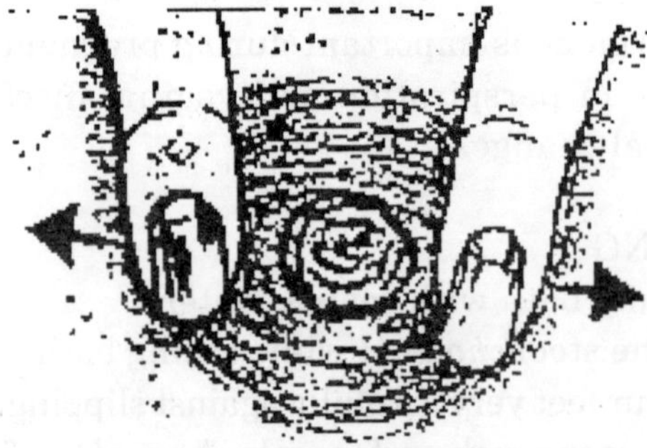

Fig. 9

4. CARE OF PERINEUM

- Wash the perineal area with soap and water (from front to back).
- Change undergarments everyday.
- Wear cotton undergarments.
- Remove pubic hairs regularly throughout the pregnancy.

5. DENTAL CARE

- Brush your teeth everyday in the morning.
- Brush your teeth after dinner also.
- Use soft toothbrush.
- Avoid tooth extraction during pregnancy.

6. CLOTHING

- Wear loose and light cotton clothes [*kameez* and *salwar*].
- Wear loose undergarments.
- Tie the salwar/petticot below the umbilicus.

7. SHOES

- Wear comfortable flat/low heel shoes/*chappals* with rough sole surface.

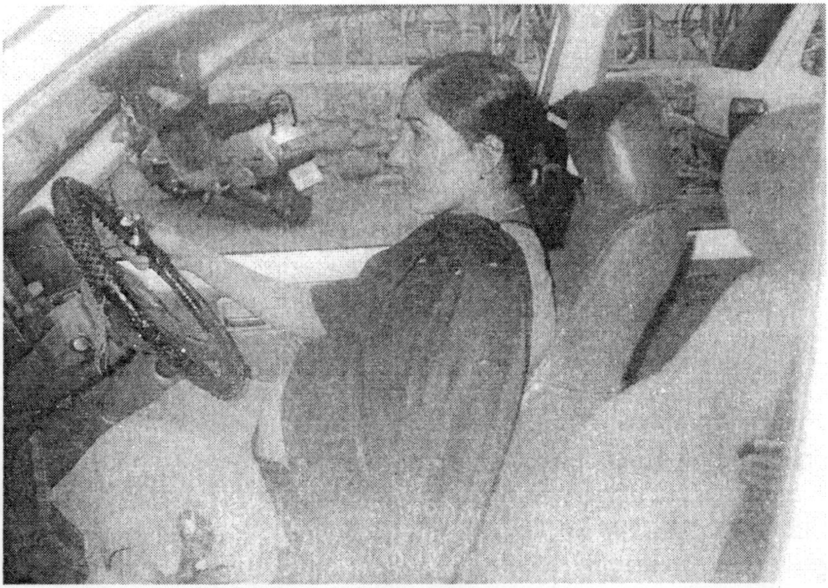

Fig. 10

8. TRAVEL

- Avoid long traveling in the 7th, 8th and 9th months of pregnancy.
- Travel in the train is more comfortable than bus.
- If you are traveling in the train walk in the train at regular intervals while holding the railings.
- *If there is bleeding p/v the traveling should be avoided.*
- If you travel in car, after every few hours take a break and walk for sometime.
- Apply seat belt with one part on the above the umbilicus and the other below the umbilicus (Fig. 10).

Do not travel in auto rickshaw.

Do not travel if there is bleeding/leakage per vagina. Go to hospital.

9. REST

- Rest for two hours in day time and 10 hours at night.
- Rest in lateral (right/left side; preferably left side).
- Keep one pillow under the head. Turn your body either left/ right side.
- Keep another pillow in between the knees.

10. SLEEP

- Sleep in well ventilated room.
- Lie down on hard mattress / *gadda*.
- Wear loose clothes during night.
- Sleep in right/left lateral position (preferably left side).

11. DIET

- Do not skip any food.
- Take meals in small quantity but at frequent intervals.
- Take any fruit such as apple, orange, banana 3-4 times a days.
- Take a glass of juice.
- Take at least 2 glasses of milk.
- Do include lots of green leafy vegetable e.g. spinach, *methi* for iron, fresh fruits for vitamins, jaggery for energy. Gram (*chana*)

Do not fast during pregnancy.

12. SUPPLEMENTS

- As advised by doctor.
- Take tablets of iron and folic acid and calcium per day.

- Iron tablets cause constipation and black stools.
- Take lot of fluids regularly.

13. HOUSEHOLD ACTIVITIES

A. Avoid lifting heavy objects.

B. Lift objects from the floor in following manner (Fig. 11)

- Bring the object near the body.
- Keep your back straight
- Bend your knees. Then lift the object.

C. Cleaning the floor

- Clean the floor in sitting position.

D. Cooking

- Do not cook for long time in standing position.
- Do cooking in sitting position.

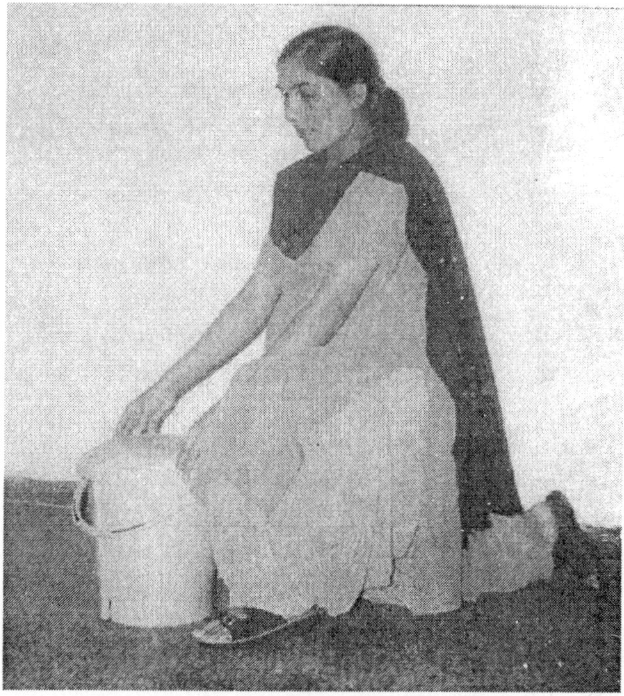

Fig. 11

14. INJECTION TETANUS TOXOID (TT)

- Have two doses of Injection T-T with a gap of 4-6 weeks between the two doses. First dose should be as early as possible.

15. COITUS

- Sexual intercourse is not prohibited in pregnancy.
- However, avoid sexual intercourse in last one and half months of pregnancy.

16. DRUGS

- Do not take any medicine without advice by doctor.

17. SMOKING

- Do not smoke during pregnancy.
- Ask the husband and the family members not to smoke in that room where you sit/sleep.

Do not sit in that environment where smoke is there.

Do not expose to X-ray and eclipse.

Do not keep fast.

18. CORRECT POSTURES

Standing

- Put equal weight on both legs.
- Keep your feet apart.
- Both abdomen and buttocks tucked in.
- Keep your shoulders relaxed at the side and down.

Sitting (Fig. 1-2)

- Choose comfortable chair
- Support your back against the back of the chair.
- Thighs should rest on the chair.
- Keep the knees slightly higher than hips.
- Keep your feet on the floor or *peedhi*.
- On easy chair, support your head with pillow and raise your legs on the stool.

Sit close to your desk / table to avoid bending forward.

19. LYING DOWN

Side – Lying Position (Fig. 4)

- Keep one pillow under the head and another under the arm.
- Straighten the lower leg.
- Flex upper leg.
- Keep one pillow under the upper leg.

Half Back Lying Position (Fig. 12)

- Keep 2-3 pillows under the head.
- Keep one pillow under the back and another under the knees.
- Straighten the legs.

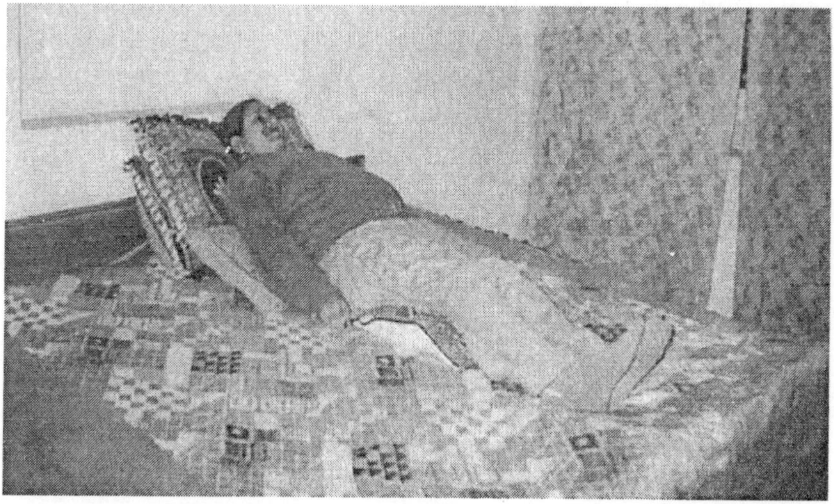

Fig. 12

Getting Up From Lying Position (Fig. 5)

- Bend your knees
- Roll on to one side.
- Put the pressure on one elbow joint to prevent strain on back and abdomen.
- Hand of another arm should touch the bed.
- Sit for 2-3 minutes, then walk if you want.

20. ANTENATAL EXERCISES

Guidelines for Exercises

- Regular exercises (at least 3 times a week)
- Stop exercise when you feel tired.
- Exercise in safe and in cool surroundings.
- Drink extra fluid before and after exercising.
- Avoid exercises with jerking, bouncing and jumping.
- Avoid any type of exercises that cause a loss of balance, falling or mild abdominal injury.

- Avoid exercises that require you to lie on your back after 3rd and 4th month of pregnancy.
- Empty your bladder before exercises.

Pelvic Tilting or Rocking Exercises

- Lie down in half lying position.
- Bend knees with feet flat on the bed / floor.
- Place one hand under the small of your back.
- Place another hand on the top of your abdomen.
- Tighten the abdomen and buttocks.
- Lift the buttocks about 3-4" from the surface.
- Press the small of the back down on to the underneath hand.
- Breathe normally, hold for up to 10 seconds than relax.
- Repeat up to 10 times.

Pelvic Floor Exercise

- Sit, stand or half lying down with legs apart.
- Close and draw up around the back passage as though preventing a bowel action.
- Repeat around the front two passages as preventing the flow of urine.
- Hold up to 10 seconds, breathing normally and relax.
- Repeat up to 10 times.

Abdominal Tightening

- Lie down in half lying position.
- Breathe in and out.
- Pull in the lower part of the abdomen below the umbilicus while breathing normally and then breathed out.
- Hold breath for 10 seconds and then relax.
- Repeat up to 10 times.

Breathing Awareness Exercises

- Sit comfortably with eyes closed.
- Take deep breath in from the nose and breath out from mouth.
- Listen to your breathing especially outward breath.
- Recognizing short pause before inward breathing naturally follows.

Foot and Leg Exercises (Fig. 13)

- Sit or half lie with back supported.
- Bend and stretch the ankles at 10-12 times.
- Circle both feet at the ankle at least 10 times in each.

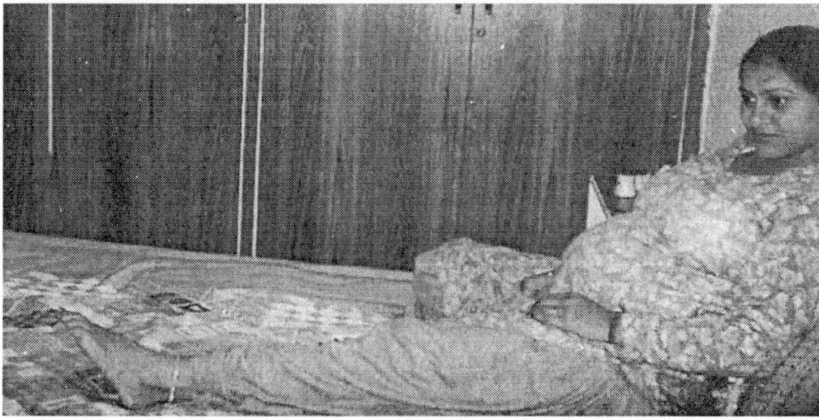

Fig. 13

Inner Thigh Stretches (Fig. 14, 15)

- Sit in a butterfly position with heels together.
- Pull the knees close to your body.
- Gently press both knees towards the floor.
- Relax.
- Repeat this for 10 times.

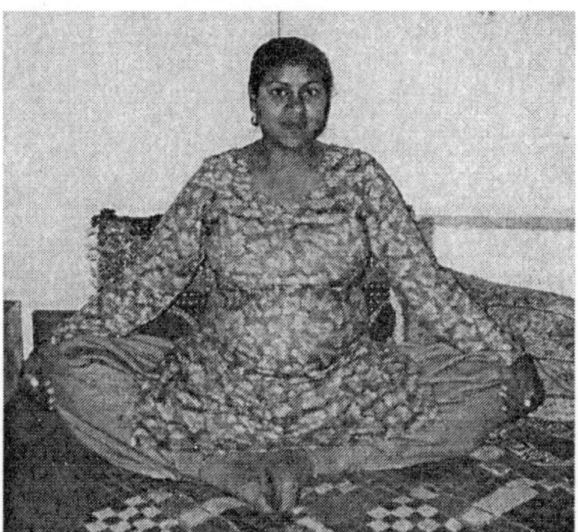

Fig. 14

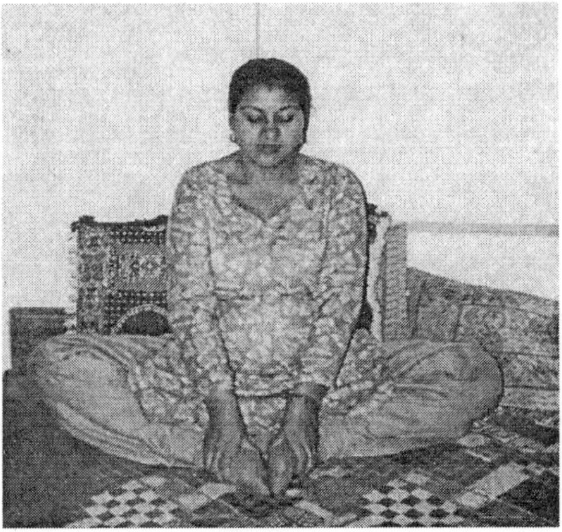

Fig. 15

Tailor Reach Exercise (Fig. 16)

- Sit with legs crossed at ankles.
- Stretch arms over head.
- Reach up with right arm, then with left arm.

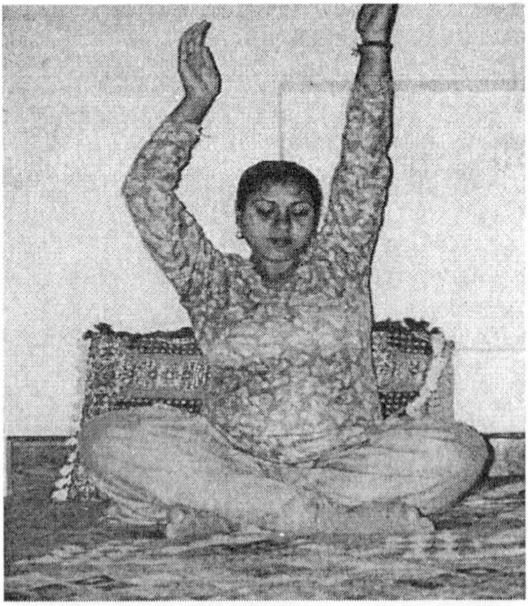

Fig. 16

Minor Disorders

DYSPNEA

- "Shortness of breath during pregnancy".

CAUSE

- Decrease in thoracic space due to the upward displacement of the diaphragm due to enlarging uterus.

DO'S	DON'TS
· Use good posture	
· Do tailor reach exercise	Overexert while doing
domestic / official activities	
· *Sleep in semi-flower position with extra pillows under the head and shoulder	
· Lie down on left lateral position	
· Eat small meals at frequent intervals	
· Consult the doctor if dyspnea is continuous	

* All position explained in self care during pregnancy.

FATIGUE AND DROWSINESS

- Feeling of weakness

DO'S	DON'TS
· Take rest, before you become overtired	Become overtired
· Take short break during the day time with your feet up	
· Eat well balanced diet (including fruits, vegetables, milk, juices etc.)	Take extra coffee
· Do exercise regularly	
· Use extra pillows for comfort during sleeping	
· Lie on left lateral side	

***HOW TO RECOGNISE ONSET OF LABOUR—SELF-CARE IN LABOUR*(AT 30-32 WEEKS PERIOD OF GESTATION)**

1. LABOUR

Labour is the process by which the baby, placenta and its membranes are expelled out through birth passage.

First Stage of Labour (Fig. 17) :- It begins with onset of time labour pains and lasts till the mouth of the womb (cervix) opens. In the first pregnancy it completed within 12 hours.

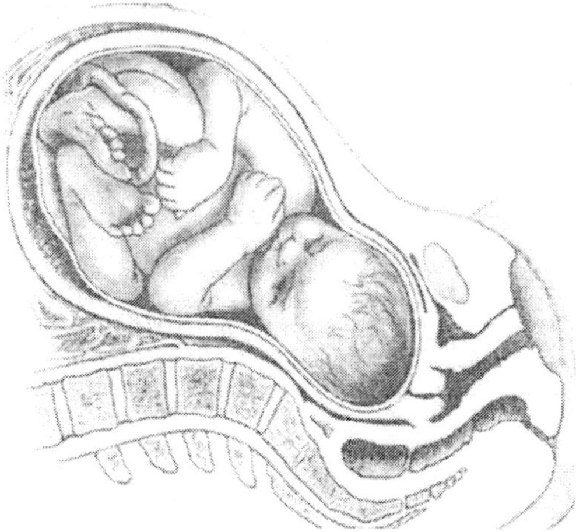

Fig. 17

Second Stage of Labour (Fig. 18) :- It begins with opening of the womb and lasts till the birth of the baby. Usually it lasts for 30-45 minutes.

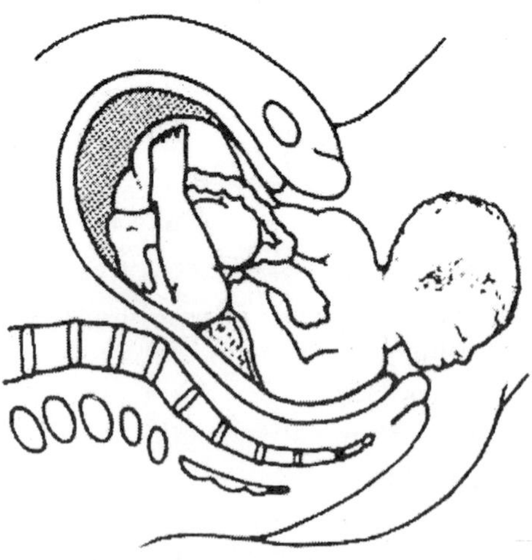

Fig. 18

Third Stage of Labour (Fig. 19) :- It lasts from the birth of the baby to coming out of placenta. It lasts for 10-30 minutes.

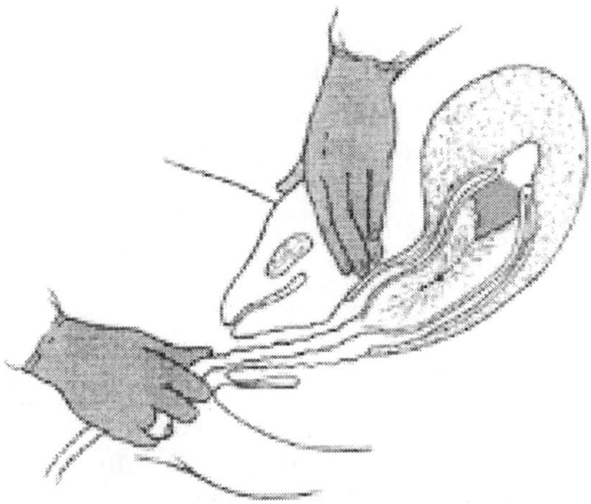

Fig. 19

2. YOUR BODY GETTING READY FOR LABOUR

a) The baby "Drops" into the pelvis (also called lightening or engagement). This can occur up to 4 weeks before labor starts.

SIGNS

- You may be able to breathe easier, but will have more pressure on your bladder.
- You feel like you need to pass urine more often.

PRELABOUR CHANGES

- You may breathe more easily.
- Increased downward (pelvic) pressure as fetus drops in the pelvis.
- Leg cramps or pains (due to pressure) may appear.
- Increased urinary frequency.
- Increased vaginal secretions.

b) A Show of Pink-Tinged Mucous (discharge or mucus plug) from your vagina may occur up to a week before your baby is born. If this looks more like blood than mucus immediately report to doctor.

c) Backache:- Backache may occur at the onset of labor. Massage, movement and bath with luke warm water will often make you feel better if your backache comes and goes in a pattern.

d) Rupture of Membranes (a gush or trickle of fluid from your vagina). It indicates that amniotic sac is leaking or broken. Immediately approach the hospital, otherwise it will cause infection.

3. RECOGNITION OF TRUE LABOUR PAINS

You should reach the hospital as soon as labour pains start. It should be differentiated from false contractions.

FALSE LABOR PAINS	TRUE LABOR PAINS
· A hardening of the abdomen without discomfort/pain.	Hardening of the abdomen with discomfort/pain.
· Pain is usually in the Abdomen/ groin/hips.	Pains begin in the back and move around the abdomen.
· Contractions are not regular, may lasts for 3-4 minutes with gap of may hours and days; not accompanied by backache.	Contractions are regular (initially of 20-30 seconds duration with interval of 10-15 minutes). Then increasing till it will be 60-90 second duration and with 1-2 minutes interval.
· Walking has no effect on false contractions. It may even lessen the false contractions.	Intensity usually increased while walking. This will help to dilate the cervix.

SELF CARE IN FIRST STAGE OF LABOUR

1. ARTICLES (To be brought during labour)

Keep the following articles ready for you and for your baby towards the end of the 9th month of pregnancy. Bring these along with you when you approach the hospital for delivery.

BASKET FOR MOTHER (Fig. 20)

- Tooth brush and paste
- Towel – small & big
- Soap
- Two sets of your suits
- Bra and undergarments
- Glass and spoon
- Sanitary pads etc.

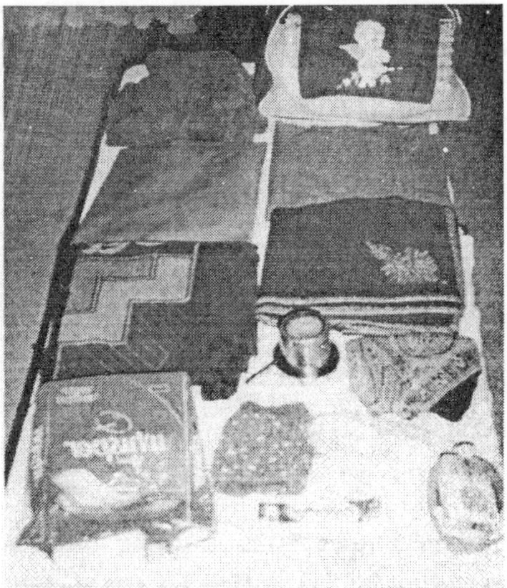

Fig. 20

BASKET FOR BABY (Fig. 21)

- Baby towel
- Baby sheet/blanket

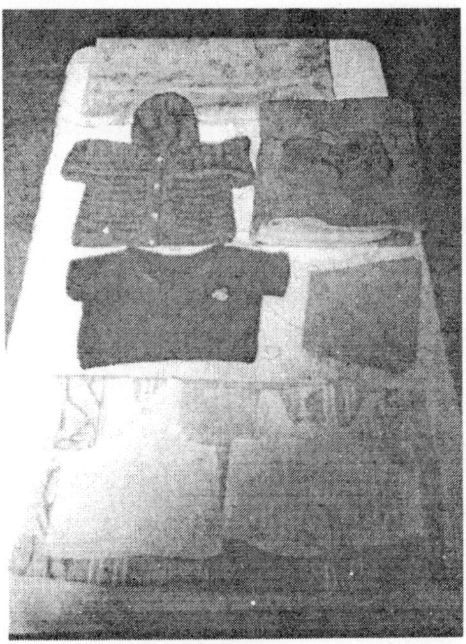

Fig. 21

- Baby napkins (5 in number made of old clean clothes)
- Under shirt
- Shirt/frock
- Cardigans in winter cap, socks
- Baby soap

2. BATH

Take bath with luke-warm water and wear clean clothes before coming to the hospital.

3. POSITION

- Adopt the position in which you feel more comfortable during contractions.
- Sit on chair/bed in early labor.
- Lie down in semidorsal, recumbent Fowler's position [head little high, left side] Do not sit on the floor

4. MOBILITY

Walk in early labor in the labor room (consult doctor). Follow doctor's advice.

5. NUTRITION

Always take fluids tea/juice/cold drinks and snacks such as biscuits/toast every 30-60 mt when labour has started contractions.

Undernourishment leads to physiological exhaustion, dehydration. This affects the fetal heart.

6. BLADDER CARE

- Empty your bladder every hourly in the toilet if there is no intravenous drip during initial uterine contractions.
- During active uterine contractions empty your bladder in the bed pan. Empty bladder helps the fetus to come down.

7. BOWEL CARE

- Bowels will be cleaned after giving enema by the nurse.
- Wash your perineal area with soap & water after enema.

8. VAGINAL EXAMINATION

Vaginal examination is essential to see the progress of the labour so you should

- Empty your bladder.
- Remove your underwear.
- Keep your buttocks near the edge of the table.
- Take deep breathe while per-vaginal examination is going on.
- Clean the perineal area and keep perineal pad. Do not touch the perineal area with your hands.

SELF CARE IN SECOND STAGE OF LABOUR

This is the stage when your baby is coming out.

1. HOW DO YOU KNOW THIS STAGE STARTED

- Expulsive uterine contraction:- During this you will feel like pushing the baby. Contractions will last 60-90 seconds with ½ minutes gap.
- During contractions you will feel that something is coming out.

2. RUPTURE OF THE FOREWATERS

You will feel there will be gush of water from the birth canal.

- Keep the perineal area clean.
- Keep the pad.

3. SHOW

More thick discharge (blood and mucus) from the birth passage.

4. DILATATION AND GAPING OF THE ANUS

- At this time cervix will be completely opened (10cm).

With the pressure of presenting part (fetus) there will be widening of the anus.

5. APPEARANCE OF THE PRESENTING-PART

- During contractions due to gaping of the vaginal canal, presenting part will be seen.

SELF-CARE

1. NUTRITION

- Take a sip of water in between since your throat may go dry due to exertion.

2. HYGIENE

- Clean your face with a small towel as there will be more sweating in this stage.

3. TRANSFER FROM BED TO DELIVERY TABLE

- As soon as you are in second stage of labor, you will be shifted from the bed to the delivery table.
- You should sit in the wheel chair i.e. on the stretcher.

4. POSITION ON THE DELIVERY TABLE

- You should come from the wheel chair/ stretcher on the delivery table.
- Keep your buttocks at the edge of table.
- Keep your feet near the delivery table poles.
- Keep your head and shoulder on the pillow.

5. WHEN TO PUSH

- You should push the baby when it is advised by the doctor/ nurse.
- Your voice will change. It will become deep.

You will feel involuntary passage of fetus

6. HOW TO PUSH THE BABY

- When contraction (pain) begins you should take 2 short deep breath and hold while pulling back on knees and pushing down abdominal muscles as you are expelling hard stool.
- Keep your jaws relaxed.
- Take deep breath and relax when the contraction is gone.

Within 30-45 minutes this stage will be over

7. EPISIOTOMY (AFTER-LOCAL ANAESTHESIA)

- Doctor/Nurse will give one injection in the perineum to anaesthetize it.
- One incision will be given on the perineum to widen the birth passage for the baby to come out.

8. SEE YOUR BABY

- As soon as baby comes out have a look at your baby.
- Ask the nurse/doctor to show the sex of the baby before cutting the cord.

SELF-CARE IN THIRD STAGE OF LABOUR

1. EXPULSION OF THE PLACENTA

- After the baby comes out, placenta will be out within 10-15 minutes.

2. SUTURING OF EPISIOTOMIES

- *Do not touch the perineum while episiotomy is being sutured* Incision which was given on the perineum will be sutured within 10-15 minutes.

3. CLEAN YOUR BODY AND CHANGE YOUR CLOTHES

- Clean your face, body and change your clothes.
- Wear bra, underwear, *kameez*, *salwar* or / blouse, petticot and *sari*.

4. NUTRITION

- Take tea and biscuits.

5. COMFORT

- Lie in lateral position (Left/Right).

6. BREAST FEEDING

- Give breast feed to your baby as soon as possible.

7. DANGER SIGNS

A number pf complications may arise in the postnatal period. It may be life threatening. If there are following danger signs, immediately see your doctor/nurse.

- Inability to pass urine.
- Severe pain at the episiotomy site.
- Fever
- Foul smelling discharge from vagina
- Abdominal pain
- Abnormal behavior
- Prolonged and profuse bleeding from genital tract.
- Painful and swollen legs.
- Painful breast/unilateral pain in breast.
- Subinvolution of uterus.

(a) SELF CARE OF MOTHER IN POSTNATAL PERIOD

SELF CARE IN POSTNATAL PERIOD

It is the post delivery period (up to 42 days / 6 weeks) when your internal system will return to a non-pregnant state.

1. CHANGES IN THE BODY

(a) CHANGES IN THE UTERUS:- This is the process of the uterus contracting to a non-pregnant size, within 10 days after delivery. It involutes about 1-2 cm per day.

LOCHIA:- Lochia is the vaginal discharge which comes out for 4-6 weeks after delivery. There are three types of lochia.

Type	*Characteristics*	*Duration*	*Quantity*
Lochia Rubra (red)	Blood tinged red discharge	3-4 days	Profuse
Lochia Serosa (pink)	Brown to yellow discharge	5-14 days	Diminishing
Lochia Alba (white)	Turbid whitish discharge	15 days to 6 weeks	Scanty

MENSTRUATION (PERIOD)

- It may start within 6-8 months or earlier after birth of your baby, when baby is on breast feeding.
- You may have your first menstrual 6-8 weeks after delivery if you are not breastfeeding your baby.
- Pregnancy can occur before your first period.
- Consult your doctor/nurse to discuss birth control option.

(b) MOOD CHANGES:- Rapid mood changes with crying or laughing for no apparent reason due to hormonal and life style changes.

EMOTIONAL CHANGES

- Feeling of sadness.
- Crying/laughing for no apparent reason
- Feel very tired
- Poor concentration

What to do:

- Rest when your baby sleeps
- Limit your visitors
- Talk to someone.

2. BATHING

- You can take bath any time after delivery. Always take bath with soap and water
- Wear clean clothes.

3. PERINEAL CARE

- Wash your perineal area with soap and warm tap water.
- Dry the perineal area.
- Keep clean cloth/ pad on perineum.
- Wear clean underwear.
- Change your underwear everyday.

4. CARE OF EPISIOTOMY SITE

- Wash the episiotomy site with soap and water during taking bath and after each voiding.
- While washing inspect for any gaping, swelling and pain on the stitches.
- Keep clean cloth/sterile pads on perineum.

DO'S	DON'TS
· Lie on your side when you rest or sleep	Rest / sleep on you back for long time
· Sit with your legs flexed	Sit with parting your legs
· Change your pads at least 5 times per day.	Keep same cloth / pad more than 3-4 hours.
	Touch the surface of your pads before using them.

Report to your doctor /nurse

- If your perineum seems very painful
- Gaping in the episiotomy site.

5. CARE OF BLADDER

- Always keep your bladder empty.
- Within 1-2 hour after the birth of your baby you should pass urine.

- Thereafter, empty your bladder at 4-6 hours interval.
- Wash the perineal area with soap and water.

DO'S	DON'TS
· Start fluid (tea, milk, water) immediately after delivery.	Practice withdrawal of fluid intake
· Go to toilet at every 4-6 hours interval to empty the bladder.	
· Report to the doctor/nurse if you failed to empty your full bladder	Hesitate to explain your condition to the doctor/ nurse.

6. CARE OF BOWEL

You can expect to have bowel movement within 3 days of your baby's birth. Prevent constipation.

DO'S	DON'TS
· Drink 6-8 glasses of fluids per day	· Restrict fluid unless doctor advises it
· Try to eat plenty of fruits vegetable and whole grains.	· Forget to contact doctor/ nurse if you feel you need to have a bowel movement but you can't; your bowel movements are painful and hard; you haven't had a bowel movement by 5 days after your baby's birth.
· You must take lot of *dal* and green leafy vegetables, spinach, *methi*, radish and drumstick leaves	

7. BREAST CARE

- While taking bath, wash your breasts with soap and water.
- Dry with clean soft towel.
- Wear bra to support the breasts (size more than 1-2 nos.)

8. NUTRITION

- You should eat more than your usual diet.
- Start normal diet within 24 hours after delivery.
- You should drink plenty of fluids like juice, soup.
- You must eat a lot of *dal*, green leafy vegetable (spinach, *methi*, *sagg*), radish, and drumstick leaves.

- You should take one tablet of iron folic acid for 100 days.

DON'T

- Take extra *ghee* in your diet
- Keep any fast till baby is on breast feed milk.

9. REST AND SLEEP

After delivery you must take rest which will help you to regain your body strength. Here are some suggestions to help you do that.

- Plan to spend a few days alone with your baby and support people before having relatives.
- Take rest or sleep when your baby sleeps (because your baby's waking and sleeping pattern may be different from yours).
- Use feeding time as a chance to rest (e.g. breast feeding while lying down).
- Ask for and accept help from friends and family such as preparing food doing house work and laundry.

DO'S	DON'TS
· Go to bed early.	Have many visitors in first week.
· Do light exercises.	Climb stairs more than necessary.
· Take rest in afternoon.	Lift heavy weight.

10. AFTER PAINS

After your baby is born your uterus will continue to contract as it returns to its original shape and size these are normal contractions of the uterus and should fade after the first few days postpartum.

- Place a warm water bottle on your abdomen.
- Relaxation breathing exercises.

11. POST PARTUM EXERCISES

· The aim of postpartum exercise is to improve the muscle tone which are stretched during pregnancy and labor (especially the abdominal and perineal muscles).

When to start :

- In normal vaginal delivery with episiotomy – after 15 days.
- In caesarean section – after 6 weeks.

EXERCISES

Points to be remember

- Empty your bladder before exercises.
- Use flat surface for exercises.

PELVIC FLOOR EXRCISES (Fig. 22, 23)

- You should contract the pelvic muscles in a manner to withhold the act of defecation or urination and then relax.
- These exercises can be performed during everyday activities such as feeding, bathing, nappy changing and after each bladder- emptying.
- During exercise contractions should be held for 10 seconds.

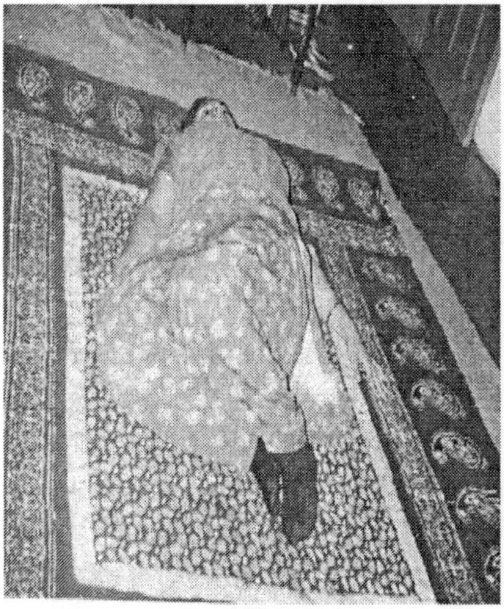

Fig. 22

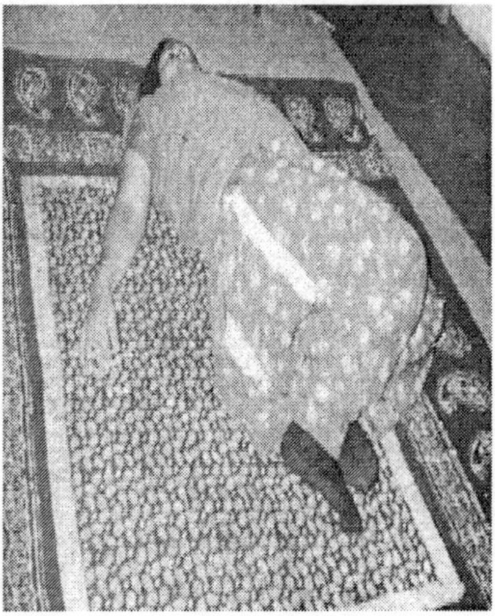

Fig. 23

KNEE ROLLING

- Lie down on back with knees bent.
- Pull in the abdomen and roll both knees to one side as far as comfortable.
- Keep shoulders flat.
- Return knees to an upright position and relax the abdomen.
- Repeat it on other side.
- Perform this exercise up to 10 times.

HIP HITCHING (Fig. 24)

- Lie down in the back
- Bent one knee and
- Straighten the other knee

- Slide the heel of the straight leg downwards thus lengthening the leg
- Shorten the same leg by drawing the hip up toward the ribs on same side.
- Repeat up to 10 times, keeping the abdomen pulled in.
- Change to the opposite side and repeat it.

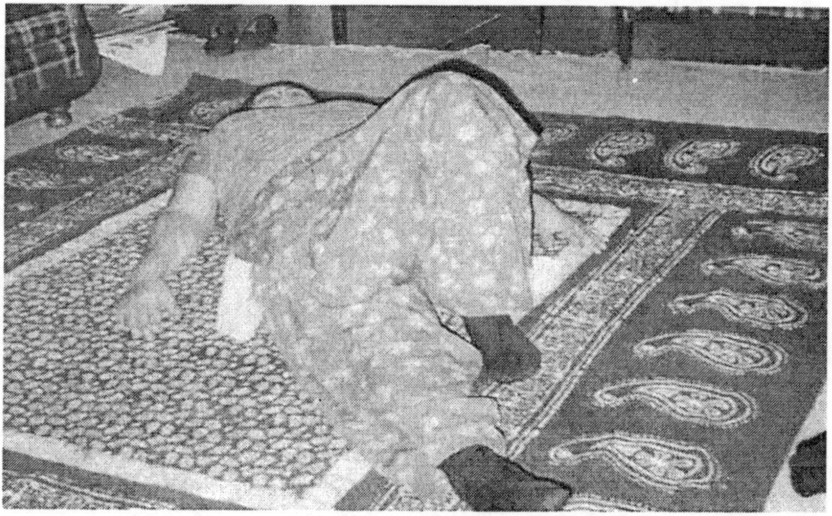

Fig. 24

SEXUALITY AND HEALTHY RELATIONSHIPS

The time to restart sexual relations is

- When you are physically comfortable.
- When both of you feel emotionally ready.
- Talking about your feelings may help to understand each other's need.
- You can express your sexuality in many ways (intimacy and caring for one another such as cuddling, hugging, kissing.)

FOLLOW UP

- Come in postnatal clinic after 6 weeks for check-up, and counseling for family planning.

12. BIRTH CONTROL

- Space your family upto three years.
- Have a copper 'T' for 5 years.
- Condom can be used.

Do not use Oral Pills till your breast feed your baby

b) CARE OF THE BABY

1. BREAST FEEDING

Breast milk is one of the most precious gifts you give to your baby

WHILE YOU ARE IN HOSPITAL

- Keep your baby with you.
- Breastfeed your baby during the day and night.

BREAST AND NIPPLE CARE

- Always handle your breast with clean hands.
- Bathe as usual.
- After breast feeding leave a drop of colostrums/milk on your nipples. (Helps to prevent infection and lubricate your nipples).
- Wear proper fitting bra.

THERE IS NO NEED TO WASH YOUR BREASTS EVERY TIME BEFORE FEEDING YOUR BABY

WHEN TO BREAST FEED & FOR HOW LONG

You should put the baby on your breast when she/he

- Show signs of hunger.
- Before your baby begins to cry.
- Completely empty one breast before putting the baby to second breast.

BREAST CHANGES

After birth your breast will become larger, heavier and possibly tender as they start producing more milk

WHEN YOUR BREASTS ARE FULL YOU CAN RELIEVE THIS BY (Fig. 25-28)

- Applying heat to your breasts with warm, moist towel or a warm water bath, just before breast-feeding.

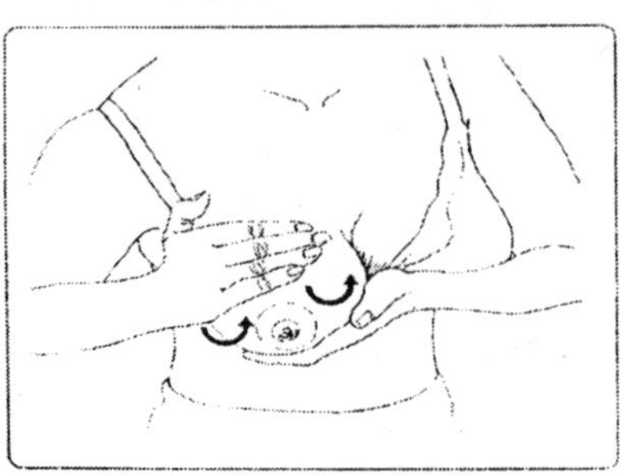

Fig. 25

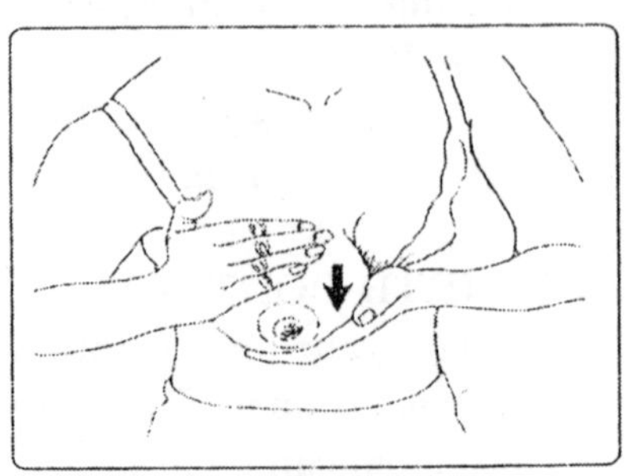

Fig. 26

- Massaging gently from the top of your breast toward your nipple to help your milk flow before and during breast-feeding.
- Express some milk to soften your breast so that your baby latches easier.

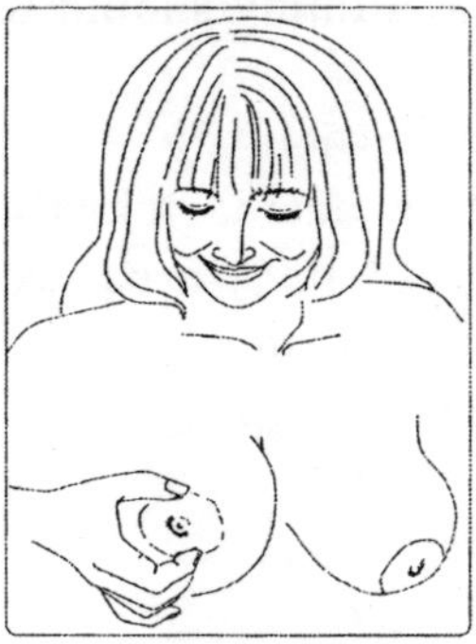

Fig. 27

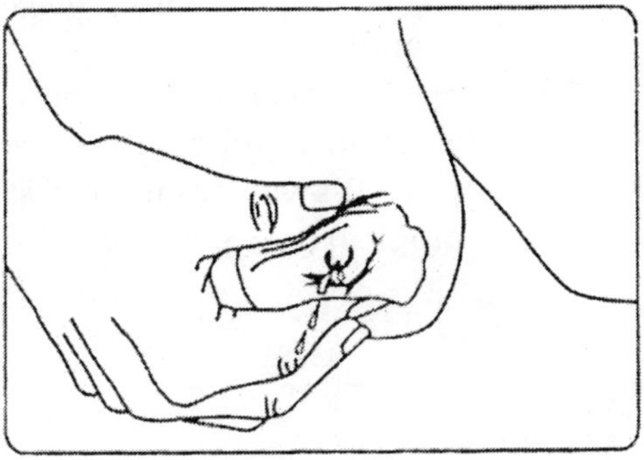

Fig. 28

HOW TO POSITION YOUR BABY WHILE BREAST FEEDING (Fig. 29-32)

Babies feed best when they are quiet and alert.

- Support your back by using pillows and feet on a stool.
- Hold your baby so she/he is lying on one side facing your breast and tucked close to your body.

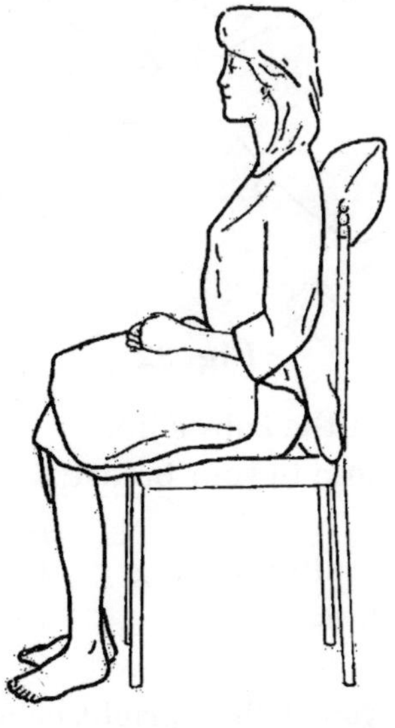

Fig. 29

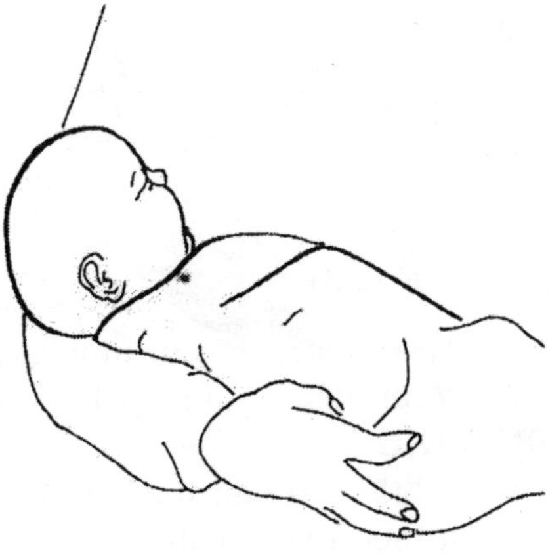

Fig. 30

IF YOUR BABY IS SLEEPY AT THE BREAST, YOU CAN KEEP YOUR BABY AWAKE BY STROKING THE BABY'S BODY OR BY GENTLY MASSAGING YOUR BREAST.

- Your arms support baby's body. Baby tummy should touch your tummy.
- Keep her/his head in between your elbow joint.
- With another hand hold your breast by placing your thumb on top, well away from your areola (the dark area around your nipples) [see pictures of different positions].

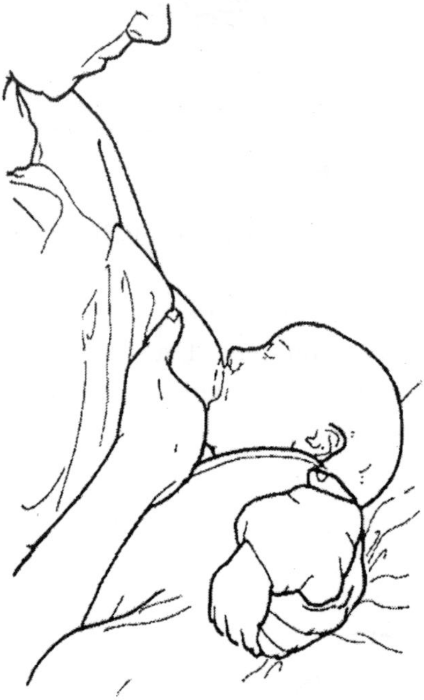

Fig. 31

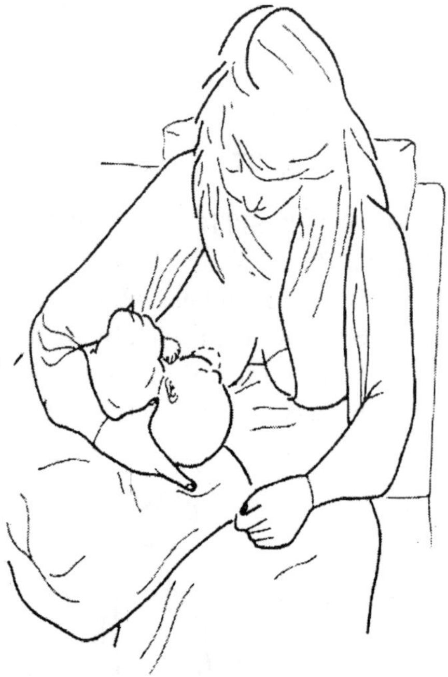

Fig. 32

- Gently stroke your nipple against the baby's lips.
- Your baby's chin needs to stay close to your breast.

BURPING

To expel the gas / air bubbles during or after feeding.

- Support your baby's chest and chin.
- Gently rub/pat your baby's back.
- Use different positions holding your baby upright or across you lap (Fig. 33).

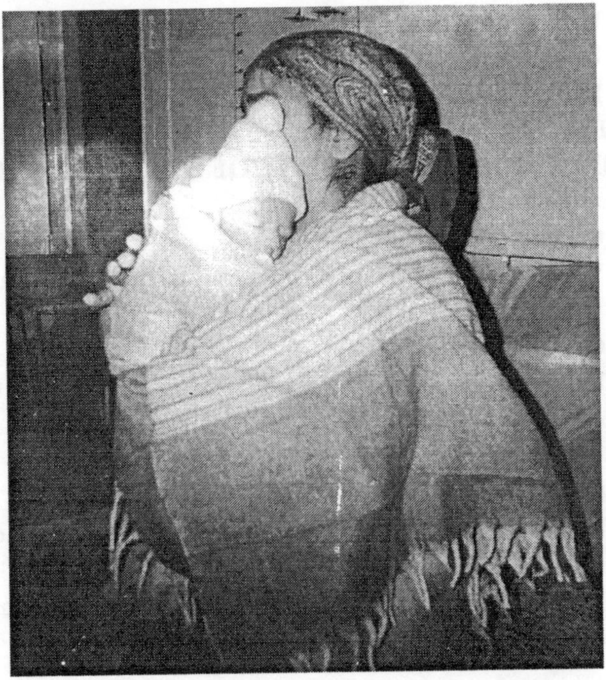

Fig. 33

2. MASSAGE

- Begin by making tiny circles on the baby's head, then smoothen the baby's forehead, jaw.
- With both hands at the centre of the baby gently press outward.
- Rubbing the hand to warm them, stroke the baby's chest.
- Stroke each arm alternating your two hands from centre outwards; open and massage each finger of each hand.
- Massage the tummy, one hand following the other, from the baby's right side to the left in a clock-wise direction.
- Stroke each leg between the two hands. Massage each foot.
- Stroke the baby's back.
- Stroke the buttocks in a circular motion.

3. CARE OF EYES

Use a clean wet swab (boil and cool it) wipe from the inner corner to the outer corner of the eye.

- Wash your hands with soap and water.
- Use one swab for one stroke.
- Do not use any *kajal / surma* in his/her eyes.

GO TO THE DOCTOR IF YOUR BABY'S EYES ARE REDDENED OR HAVE A LOT OF STICKY DISCHARGE

4. CARE OF MOUTH

Wipe your baby's mouth with clean soft wash cloth everyday.

5. CARE OF NAILS

Use only small blunt scissors (not pointed) to cut the finger and toe nails.

6. BATHING

Baby need to bathed daily (depends upon the condition of the baby). (see Photographs)

- Talking calmly to your baby will reassure your baby that all is well.

STEPS

Check the temperature of the water with your wrist/elbow.

- Apply a small amount of baby oil after the bath if baby skin is dry.
- Clean/wash the head of the baby first.
- Clean the baby face (Don't apply soap on the face).
- Keep the baby on the table / bed in the towel.
- Remove the towel, apply soap on whole body.
- Hold baby-keeping head upwards.
- Keep the baby body in the water tub.
- Remove whole soap from the body by pouring water.

NEVER POUR WATER ON THE HEAD AND FACE DIRECTLY

7. CARE OF UMBLICAL CORD

Keep the cord area dry to promote healing.

- A small amount of oozing or bleeding is normal when the cord is ready to fall off.
- Clean cord after the bath with spirit swabs.

Approach your doctor if your baby's cord area
- Has lot of blood
- Is red, warm or swollen.
- Has a foul- smelling discharge.
- Is very wet.

DON'T APPLY ANY OIL / *GHEE* ON THE CORD AREA

8. BABY'S CLOTHING

Clothes for baby should be
- Large enough for your baby to feel comfortable.
- Use cotton clothes.
- Easy to put on.
- Don't over-dress your baby.
- Use always front open shirt with buttons.
- Avoid small buttons.
- Wash all new and old clothes with mild soap and dry it under the sun but never let them dry on the ground.

9. CARE OF BOWEL / BLADDER

Baby will pass black, sticky stools called meconium within first 48 hours of delivery.
- Baby will pass urine within 24 hours after birth.
- Keep the perineal area clean and dry.

No. of diapers soiled by the baby as per frequency of breastfeeding		
Days	Breast feed per day	Wet diapers per day
First 24 hours	Offer every 3 hours	Minimum-1
Day 2	Increasing of feeds	Minimum-2
Day 3	8-12 times in 24 hour	Minimum-3
Day 4	8-12 times in 24 hour	Minimum-4
After 4 days	8-12 times in 24 hour	Increasing number of heavy wet diapers. (6 or more)

10. CARE OF BABY'S PERINEAL AREA AND DIAPERS

- Wash your hands
- Place your baby on safe, flat surface.
- Remove the soiled or wet diaper.

- Dry your baby's diaper carefully under the sun.
- Dispose off the used diaper and wash your hands.
- Clean the perineal area with wet cotton swabs/wash the perineal area.
- For baby girl wipe gently from front to back.
- A baby boy's penis is covered by skin (foreskin)

DO NOT PULL THE FORESKIN BACK FORCEFULLY

11. COMMON PROBLEMS OF NEW BORN

Most of babies following problems but can lead to major problems. So always contact your doctor if there is

- Not accepting feed
- Jaundice
- Head shape during birth little change in the shape head due to caput formation. do not message on the head.
- Excessive crying
- Diarrhea
- Constipation
- New born-rash
- Sneezing
- Vomiting
- Fever / hypothermia
- Diaper rash

34

Prolapse Uterus

Santosh Kumari and AJ Singh

Introduction:

Uterine prolapse is one of the most common gynecological conditions in India. It results from stresses of child bearing due to stretched and weakened support to the uterus. Further damage by repeated pregnancies may be the precipitating factor resulting in distressing and occasionally disabling prolapse of uterus. It is the most unfortunate scene to witness a woman with uterus hanging between the thighs affecting her mental state because of the disability which may be associated with it e.g. vaginal discharge, with occasional blood stains from the ulcer[1, 2]

Definition: Uterine prolapse is the descent of the uterus into the vagina below its normal anatomic position. In severe cases bladder may also descend pressing against the anterior or posterior vaginal wall. Uterine prolapse descent is classified into 4 categories:

First degree: Descent of cervix in the vagina.

Second Degree: Descent of cervix into the vaginal opening

Third Degree: Descent of the cervix outside the vaginal opening.

Fourth Degree (Procidentia): Permanent descent of the whole uterus below vaginal opening [3-4].

Prevalence: In India 5-18% of all women suffer from prolapsed uterus [5-8]. It constitutes a sizeable proportion of all gynecological admissions. Among nulliparous women incidence of 5-8 % has been reported.[9] Congenital uterine prolapsed has also been reported.[10]

Sign and Symptoms: The symptoms of prolapse are relieved by rest and their severity depends upon each individual patient (i.e., some women are not much bothered by even severe degree of prolapse while others complain of more botheration with mild degree of prolapse). The symptoms are:

- Something coming out of vagina.[3,7,8,11-13]
- A sensation of fullness (a peculiar foreign body sensation) in the vagina.It may be noted that a similar sensation is felt in severe vaginitis also.[3,7,8,11-13]
- A dragging sensation or discomfort or a bearing down sensation in the lower abdomen. [3,7,8,11-13]
- Low backache. [3,7,8,11-13]
- Urinary symptoms: frequent urge to pass urine, stress incontinence, difficulty in passing urine and need to reduce the mass with fingers to empty the bladder.[3,7,8,11-13]
- Repeated attack of dysuria, urinary frequency . [3,7,8,11-13]
- Urinary infection due to organisms invading the retained pool of urine.[7,8,11-13]
- Vaginal discharge.[3,7,8,11-13]
- Lax vagina, with little or no sensation during intercourse. [3,7,8,11-13]
- A discharge or bleeding caused by ulceration of dependent portion of prolapse.[7,8,11-13]
- Excessive flow in periods (if patient is young).[7,8,11-13]
- Passing of gas/ flatus through vagina.[7,8,11-13]
- Painful sexual intercourse.[3,7,8,11-13]
- Rectal symptoms: They are not as common as urinary symptoms. Difficulty in emptying the bowel due to the load of faeces leading to bulge in the rectum. This mass also need to be compressed with fingers through vagina so that woman can pass faeces.[3,7,8,11-13]

Risk factors: the principal cause of prolapse is the failure of supporting structures, as a result of (1) obstetrical trauma and (2) postmenopausal atrophy.

- Age and parity
  Although prolapse occasionally occurs in nulliparous women, it is most common among women who have many children. Prolapse increases with age and parity. Genital prolapse is very common in young women in India. In a study by the authors, 72% women in Chandigarh were reported to have the onset of prolapse before 30 years of age[8].
- Family history of prolapse as a predisposing factor has a significant effect on prolapse of the uterus.[13]
- Injuries related to childbirth may also precipitate prolapse, e.g.-
  1. Prolonged distension of the birth canal, as in prolonged second stage of labor[4,14]
  2. Precipitate labor as may occur in grandmultipara.[4, 14]
  3. Traction on the presenting part of the baby before the cervix is fully dilated, as it occurs in vaccum extraction and forceps delivery. Premature bearing down before full dilatation of cervix results in overstretching of pelvic floor muscles[13-14]
  4. Pressure exerted on abdomen to deliver placenta.[13.]
  5. Home delivery conducted by traditional birth attendants (Dais) is another cause of prolapse. Women are often wrongly made to bear down before full dilatation of cervix, when bladder is not empty. In such cases there is undue stretching of pelvic floor muscles as episiotomy is not given by dais. Prolonged bearing down in the second stage of labour and downward vigorous push on the uterus to deliver baby and to expel placenta may weaken the ligámentary support to genital tract. Rapid successions of pregnancies preclude proper puerperal rehabilitation. In such women there is a tendency to develop prolapse.[14] One badly conducted delivery is sufficient to precipitate prolapse.[13]
  6. Delivery of big baby leads to stetching the perineal muscles leading to patulous introitus and subsequently to prolapse.[13, 14]
  7. Excessive straining in the immediate postpartum period and lack of post partum rest predispose women to prolapse.[13]

• Post menopausal atrophy: Once the women sustain injuries in their pelvic area due to repeated deliveries with resultant devitalization of the supporting tissue, the seed for prolapse is sown. Postmenopausaly, as a result of oestrogen deficiency, there is further atrophy in the supporting tissues and descent of uterus becomes inevitable.[4,13,14]

Aggravating factors: Factors which tend to aggravate uterine descent, once there is musculo-fascial weakness of the pelvic floor, such as chronic cough, constipation, obesity, lifting heavy weight are of etiological importance[13, 14]

Treatment: For the established cases of prolapse, either palliative or surgical treatment is required. Patients with varying degree of uterovaginal prolapse and posthysterectomy vaginal prolapse of different etiologies and varying degrees of symptoms may be managed according to the following choices and options, depending on a variety of individual circumstances.[15]

Management of Uterine Prolapse: Most patients who have mild degree of uterovaginal or posthysterectomy vaginal prolapse may have no or mild symptoms. Under these circumstances, surgical repair is not indicated. The patient should be informed of her condition and of associated problems that could make her condition worse (e.g. chronic cough, obesity, chronic constipation). Measures to prevent or correct these associated problems should be instituted.

The pelvic muscles provide most of the support to pelvic organs. Patients should be taught the technique of perineal muscle exercises and encouraged to do them assiduously. Periodic examination is required, and it is essential to reinforce the patient‘s motivation to continue the preventive measures. It is hoped that such an approach will prevent the need for further surgery.[15] It has been proved in randomized clinical trials that pelvic floor exercises are helpful in strengthening these muscles, which supports pelvic organs. These exercises had a success rate of 50-90% in alleviating the symptoms of prolapse.[16-18.]

Asymptomatic prolapse does not need any treatment. Symptomatic prolapse can be treated conservatively or surgically depending on the individual. Although pelvic muscle exercises may be of benefit to women with stress incontinence by strengthening urethral support, these have not proven beneficial for patients with significant prolapse. Pelvic muscle exercises are virtually never harmful, but they are not helpful in complete prolapse or procidentia[14,15]

Conservative treatment is indicated for:

(a) The patient with mild /minor degree of prolapse.

(b) Young women with reproductive ambitions.

(c) Elderly women who are poor operation risk.

(d) Antenatal and postnatal patients.

(e) Women who refuse surgery.

(f) Patients awaiting surgery, particularly when bedsores are present[14,15].

(g) Conservative management of prolapse consists of insertion of a **flexible ring pessary** as a support so that ring takes up the lateral and longitudinal slack of the vaginal wall. Ring pessaries are made of polyethylene and these are of various sizes. A size is selected that it should not cause discomfort nor be expelled from the vagina on straining. Disadvantages of the pessaries are vaginitis, vaginal discharge, pressure necrosis, vaginal necrosis, chronic irritation and erosion of pessary into bladder creating a vesico vaginal fistula.[14,15.] Patients using pessaries should get themselves examined on regular basis. Some pessaries, such as silicone doughnut pessaries can be left in place for months at a time without removal. Other pessaries ideally should be removed by the patient at bedtime each night and replaced in the morning to avoid erosions. At the initial fitting, the patient should be encouraged to insert and remove the pessary herself. If the pessary fits well and the patient is comfortable, it is helpful to reexamine her within one week and 4-6 months thereafter[15].

Surgical Management

This involves removal of the uterus (Vaginal/abdominal hysterectomy).[15]

Surgical correction of uterine descent and vaginal laxity is considered for majority of patients and, in general offers a high rate of cure, with low morbidity and mortality.[14,15.]

Patients continue to tolerate problems for years together; particularly in India, women continue to tolerate their problem for long time due to 'culture of silence 'and fatalistic attitude regarding their reproductive health problems. In two studies from north India on prolapse of uterus it was reported that majority of women had the problem for more than five years. [7, 8]

What should one do when uterine prolapse is noticed?

Once you feel you have some symptoms get examined by a gynecologist. In the initial stage simple pelvic floor exercises can be of help. But as the disease progresses it can lead to complete prolapse and ulcer formation. Do not get internal examination done by untrained/ unqualified people (e.g.), this can lead to infection.

Prevention of prolapse:

1. Early marriage and delivery at a young age is a risk factor for prolapse. Do not get girls married before 18 years of age At the first delivery mother should not be less than 20 years of age.
2. Adopt small family norm i.e. 2 child norm since multiparity also predisposes to prolapse.
3. Have good nutrition during pregnancy, regular check up during pregnancy is a must.
4. Delivery should be conducted in a hospital by a trained doctor/ nurse. Because one badly conducted delivery is sufficient to precipitate prolapse.
5. Do not bear down before cervix is fully dilated, the person conducting your delivery will ask you to bear down when needed.
6. Take adequate rest during postnatal period, avoidance of heavy domestic work, avoid lifting heavy weight and maintain abstinence for at least one and half month.
7. Regular pelvic floor exercises will help you in maintaining strong pelvic floor. Maintain ideal body weight. Avoid constipation eat healthy high fiber diet. Take plenty of fluids (1.5-2 liter) per day.
8. Adopt contraceptive methods to avoid unwanted pregnancy.

References

1. WHO, measuring reproductive morbidity. Report of technical working group. W.H.O./ M.C.H./ 90.4. Division of Family Planning. WHO, Geneva. August 30-September 1, 1989: 1-39.

2. Dass GS. Reproductive morbidity; Journal of Indian Medical Association. 1995; 93: 55-57.
3. Kerker, AV.Obstetric and Gynecology in developing countries. 1st edition, Delhi, Allied publishers 1985 : 302-303.
4. Hawkins J. Gordon B, Shaw's text book of Gynaecology. 10th edition, Delhi B.I Churchill Livingstone Pvt Ltd. 1991: 352-367
5. Lata P, Gupta T, Sood. A. Leforts' easy approach to genital prolapse in elderly. Indian Medical Gazette 1995; 129:33-34.
6. Naik K, Ahuja M, Kaduskar N, Gaikwad S,Are the trends in genital prolapse changing. Journal of Obstetric and Gynecology of India. 1993; 43: 426-431.
7. Singh A, Arora AK. Effect of uterine prolapse on the lives of rural north Indian women. Singapore Journal of Obstetric and Gynecology.2003; 34:52-58.
8. Kumari S, Walia IJ. and Singh AJ. Self reported uterine prolapse in a resettlement colony of North India. Journal of Midwifery and Women's Health.2000; 45: 343-350
9. Purandare VN. The abdominal cervicopraxy and sling operation for prolapse: A reappraisal. Journal of Obstetric and Gynecology of India. 1987; 37: 2 pages.
10. Dawn CS. Practical highlights of Genital Prolapse. Journal of Obstetric and Gynecology of India. 1998; 48: 211-215.
11. Dutta DK, Dutta. B, Surgical management of genital prolapse in an industrial hospital. Journal of Indian Medical Association 1994; 92: 366-367.
12. Wren BG, Lobo R.A. A handbook of Obstetric and Gynaecology.3rd edition London, Chapman and Hall Ltd. 1989 :330-332.
13. Sharma S., Walia I., Singh A. A case control study on uterine prolapse in a Chandigarh Slum. Bulletin PGIMER, 2003; 37: 143-48
14. Singh SRN. Text book of clinical gynecology, 1st edition, Kingston, United Co-operative printers Ltd. 1983: 108-113.
15. Thompson JD. Surgical correction in defects in pelvic organ support. In TeLinde's operative Gynecology, 8th edition Rock JA .Thompson JD. Editors, Philladelphia .Lippincott Raven publishers. 1997:951-968.
16. Wyman J., Fantl J.A., McClish D.K., Bump R.C. Comparative efficacy of behavioural intervention in the management of female urinary incontinence. Am J Obstetric and Gynecology, 1998; 179: 999-1007.

17. Markved S., Bo. K. The effect of post-natal exercises to strengthen the pelvic floor muscle. Acta Obst Gynecol Scand, 1996; 75: 382-85.
18. Morkved S., Bo. K., Schei. B., Salvesen. K.A. Pelvic muscle training during pregnancy to prevent urinary incontinence: A single-blind randomized controlled trial. Obstetric Gynecology, 2003; 101: 131-39.

35

Skin Problems of Women

Amrinder J Kanwar, Savita Yadav and Sunil Dogra

Our skin is the largest and of course the most visible organ in the body. Skin problems can have a huge impact on one's emotional well-being and stress levels. This stress can in turn aggravate the problem. Innumerable internal and external factors lead to some of the common skin problems of women. Gaining an insight into them will help us to manage the problems as well as protect the skin in a better way. Many people try to self-treat skin problems, using a range of different products. This chapter describes the common skin problems of women which may appear to be innocuous but at times can lead to great emotional and or physical distress in females. Also, brief mention is made about their prevention and non-medicinal management.

SOME COMMON SKIN PROBLEMS

1. Acne (Whiteheads and Blackheads)
2. Sun burn
3. Freckles
4. Dry skin
5. Melasma

6. Cracked feet
7. Stretch marks
8. Dark under eye circles
9. Allergy to artificial jewellery
10. Sun tanning
11. Enlarged Pores
12. Wrinkles
13. Cellulite

HAIR PROBLEMS

1. Dandruff
2. Hair fall
3. Greying of hair

NAIL PROBLEMS

1. Brittle nails
2. Paronychia

SOME COMMON SKIN PROBLEMS :

ACNE

Acne is a common skin problem of people in their teenage years to early adulthood, usually starting at the onset of puberty. It is most common on the face, but can also occur on the neck, chest, back, shoulders, scalp, and upper arms and legs. Aside from scarring, its main effects are psychological, such as reduced self-esteem.

It is caused by changes in the pilosebaceous units (skin structures consisting of a hair follicle and its associated sebaceous glands). Acne develops as a result of blockages in follicles. Typical acne lesions are comedones, inflammatory papules, pustules and nodules. Hyperkeratinization and formation of a plug of keratin and sebum (a microcomedo) is the earliest change. Enlargement of sebaceous glands and an increase in sebum production occur with increased androgen (DHEA-S) production at adrenarche. The microcomedo may enlarge to form an open comedo (blackhead) or closed comedo (whitehead).

WHITEHEADS

These are caused by the accumulation of hardened sebum or oil in the pores of the skin. They appear in the form of tiny, pearly, white raised spots. It occurs when a plug of sebum blocks a hair follicle deeper in the skin.

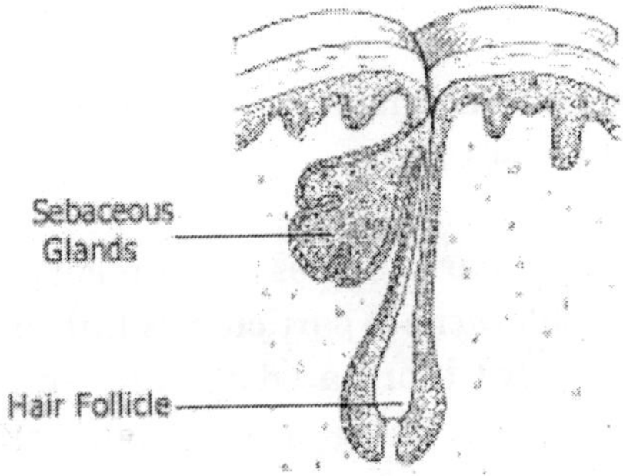

Healthy Skin

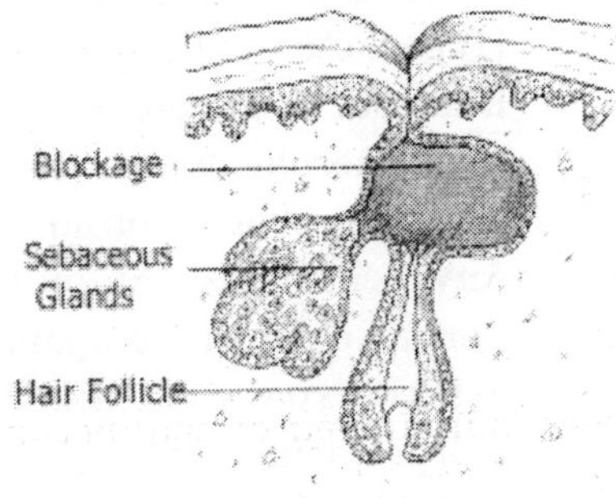

Whitehead

BLACKHEADS

A blackhead results when dead skin cells and sebum block a hair follicle near the surface of the skin. The mixture of pigment (the protein that gives skin its color) from the dead skin cells and sebum makes a blackhead dark; it is not dirt that can be washed away. Blackhead causes the pores to be further enlarged and women with oily skin end up with a skin texture that is course and rough.

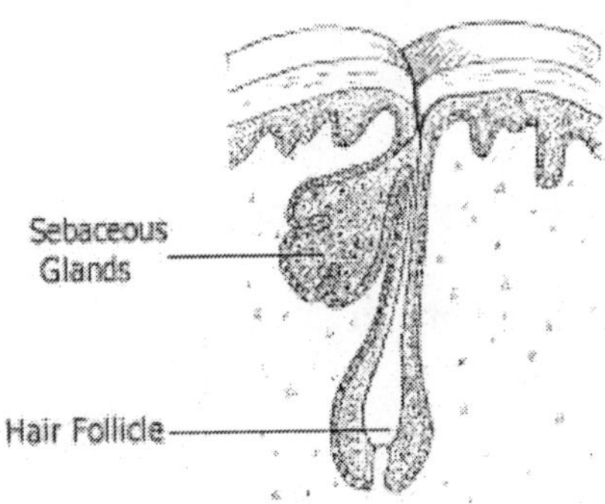

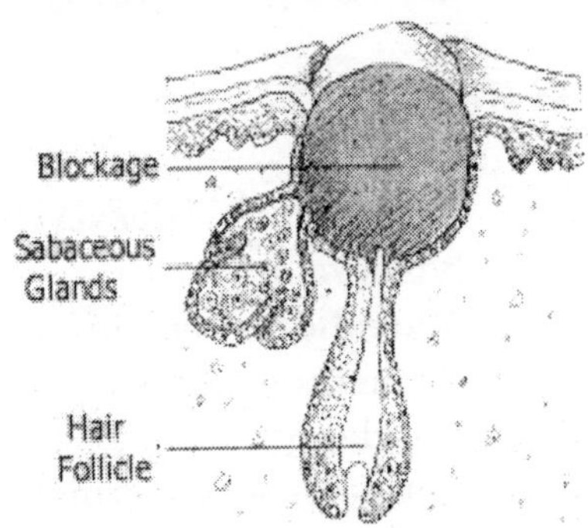

Why only some people get acne is not fully known. It is known to be partly hereditary but several other factors are known to be linked to acne:

- Family/Genetic history.
- Hormonal activity – at puberty, an increase in male sex hormones called androgens cause the glands to get larger and make more sebum.

- Stress, through increased output of hormones from the adrenal (stress) glands.
- Hyperactive sebaceous glands.
- Bacteria in the pores - Propionibacterium acnes (P. acnes) is the anaerobic bacterium that causes acne.
- Use of anabolic steroids.
- Any medication containing lithium, barbiturates or androgens.
- Certain chemical compounds – Chloracne is particularly linked to toxic exposure to dioxins, namely Chlorinated dioxins. And halogen acne is linked to exposure to halogens (e.g. iodides, chlorides, bromides).
- Diet- It has been suggested that there is a link between diets high in refined sugars and processed foods and acne.

Available treatments

Topical

1. Retinoids – Tretinoin, Adaplene, Isotretinoin, Tazarotene.
2. Antibiotics – erythromycin, clindamycin, clarithromycin.
3. Benzoyl peroxide
4. others - Azaleic acid, Nicotinamide, sulfur, salicylic acid, dapsone gel, hydroxy acids

Systemic

1. Antibiotics –

a) Tetracyclins – doxycyclin, oxytetracyclin, minocyclin, lymecyclin
b) Macrolides – erythromycin, azithromycin
c) Trimethoprim/cotrimoxazole
d) Clindamycin

3. Retinoids – isotretinoin
4. Hormonal therapy
5. Others – vit A, oral zinc, dapsone, clofazimine

Care at home (Do's and Don'ts)

(A) Regular deep pore cleansing at home and washing the face twice a day with a medicated soap and lukewarm water to reduce the oiliness of the skin surface, so as to eliminate chances of infection.

(B) Comedones should never be removed forcibly.

(C) Aim at consuming adequate amount of fruits and vegetables in your daily diet.
(D) Drink plenty of water and fresh fruit juices.
(E) Rinsing with plain water as often as possible will keep the skin free of environmental pollutants.
(F) Do not use oil-based moisturizers.

SUN BURN

Sunburn results from too much sun or sun-equivalent exposure. Almost everyone has been sunburned or will become sunburned at some time. Anyone who visits a beach, works in the yard, or simply is out in the sun can get sunburn. Although seldom fatal, sunburn can be disabling and cause quite a bit of discomfort.

Sunburn is caused by ultraviolet (UV) radiation in sun rays. The consequence is skin injury and inflammation which can start within 30 minutes of exposure. Both UVA and UVB are responsible for sunburn. Light skinned and fair-haired people are at greater risk of sunburn injury. Prior recent sun exposure and prior skin injury are risks for sunburn, even in limited exposure to the sun.

Home care starts before sunburn. If one is prepared well before going out in the sun, she won't get the burn itself. When ever one gets sunburn, the **immediate self-care is aimed at stopping the further UV radiation exposure.**

Conditions that should motivate to go to a hospital's emergency department include the following:

- Severe skin pain

Severe blistering

- Headache
- Confusion
- Nausea or vomiting
- Fainting

For mild sunburn, one may do cold compresses for 15-20 minutes. Apply aloe based lotions. Cool (not ice cold) baths may help. Avoid bath salts, oils, and perfumes because these may produce sensitivity reactions. Avoid scrubbing the skin or shaving the skin. Use soft towels and don't rub. Use a light, fragrance-free skin moisturizer or apply silver sulfadiazine. Medications such as aspirin, ibuprofen, and naproxen are useful, especially when started early. Obviously, stay out of the sun while one is sunburned.

If sunburn is moderate to severe, oral steroid therapy may be prescribed for several days. Steroid creams placed on the skin show minimal to no benefit. Stronger pain-relieving medication may be needed.

If sunburn is life threatening and you are dehydrated, then patient needs hospitalization and IV fluids or may be transferred to the hospital's burn unit.

The best prevention is to avoid the sun. This is often not practical or desired many times. Other, more practical strategies include wearing wide-brimmed hats, long-sleeved shirts, and long pants. If this is not possible, a variety of sun-blocking agents are available for use.

Pay attention to the sun protection factor (SPF). SPF is actually a ratio of the time it takes to produce a skin reaction on protected and unprotected skin. Sunscreen should be applied in generous amounts in layers and reapplied after being exposed. Activities such as sweating and swimming degrade its effectiveness.

FRECKLES

Freckles are tiny black spots spread all over the face. They tend to appear more on the areas-like the nose, cheek bones and forehead.

Our skin has its own protective mechanism against sunlight. The exposure to UV-B radiation activates melanocytes to increase the melanin production, and in those who are geneticallly predisposed it causes freckles to appear, which become more darker and numerous with continued sun exposure .

CARE:

(A) Avoid excessive exposure to sun.

(B) Use a sunscreen whenever you move out in the sun with SPF of 15 or higher.

(C) Consult a dermatologist

Although they do not need to be treated, but as some women find them unattractive they might choose to have them lightened by -

1. Medicines- retinoids, depigmenting agents
2. Electrocautery
3. Chemical peeling (spot peel or whole face peel)
4. Laser therapy (treatment using high energy beams of light).

In rare cases, they may be early changes that could lead to most serious form of skin cancer, malignant melanoma.

DRY SKIN

Dry skin is a common problem. It happens more often in the winter when cold air outside and heated air inside because of low humidity. It is more severe on lower legs, arms, flanks (sides of the abdomen), and thighs. Ordinary dry skin (xerosis) usually isn't serious, but it can be uncomfortable and unsightly, creating fine lines and wrinkles.

Most dry skin is caused by environmental factors, such as:

- **Weather.** In general, skin is driest in winter, when temperatures and humidity levels drop.
- **Central heating and air conditioning.** Central heating, wood-burning stoves, space heaters and fireplaces all reduce humidity and make the skin dry.
- **Hot baths and showers.** Frequent bathing, especially in hot water and long baths, breaks down the lipid barriers in the skin.
- **Harsh soaps and detergents.** Strong soaps and detergents strip lipids from skin and impairing the barrier.
- **Thyroid disorders.** Hypothyroidism reduces the activity of sweat and oil glands, leading to rough, dry skin.
- **Alcohol and drugs.** Alcohol and caffeine cause diuresis and dehydration.
- **Age.** With age, skin tends to become drier because oil-producing glands become less active.
- **Sun exposure.** Like all types of heat, the sun dries the skin.

The symptoms most often associated with dry skin include:

- Scaling and rough skin
- Itching
- Cracks or rarely deep fissures in the skin

Dry skin that's not cared for can lead to:

- **Dermatitis (eczema).** This condition causes redness, cracking and inflammation.
- **Folliculitis.** This is an inflammation of hair follicles.

- **Cellulitis.** This is a potentially serious bacterial infection of the skin's underlying tissues that may enter the lymphatic system and blood vessels.

Treatments and drugs

Fortunately, most dry skin results from environmental factors that can be wholly or partially controlled by home care measures.

Home Care

- Keep baths or showers short.
- Use warm (not hot) water.
- Use mild cleansers or mild soaps.
- Dry your skin thoroughly but gently — pat, don't rub.
- Use bath oils and moisturizers at least daily. Thick, greasy moisturizers work best. Apply just after a bath or shower, when your skin is still damp.
- Use a humidifier if the air is dry.
- Drink plenty of water throughout the day.
- Apply cool compresses to itchy areas.
- If skin is very dry and scaly, it is recommended to use creams containing lactic acid or lactic acid and urea.

  In most cases, dry skin problems respond well to self-care measures, One should consult the dermatologist if:
- Feel itchy without a visible rash
- Dryness and itching are preventing from sleeping
- Develop open cuts or sores from scratching
- Home care measures do not relieve dryness and itching
- Chronic or severe dry skin problems for evaluation of other related conditions like ichthyosis, psoriasis, atopic dermatitis.

MELASMA

Melasma (also known as chloasma or the mask of pregnancy when present in pregnant women) is a tan or dark facial skin discoloration. Although it can affect anyone, melasma is particularly common in women.These patches often develop gradually over time. Melasma does not cause any other symptoms beyond the cosmetic discoloration.

The pathophysiology of melasma is uncertain but following factors may play role-

1. Hormones - estrogen and progesterone cause stimulation of melanocytes or pigment-producing cells to produce more melanin pigments when the skin is exposed to sun.
2. Genetic predisposition- more than 30% of patients have a family history of melasma.
3. Thyroid disease
4. Iron deficiency
5. Drugs- Phenytoin, OCP's, HRT
6. Sun exposure – Those with light brown skin types and history of intense sun exposure are more prone to develop melasma.

Melasma presents as symmetric hyperpigmented macules, which can be confluent or punctate. The macular hyperpigmentation of melasma is commonly tan to brown. Blue or black may be evident in patients with dermal melasma.

There are three patterns of distribution: centrofacial, malar, or mandibular. A rare pattern confined to the forearms is also seen in women.

Lab Studies

- Usually, no laboratory tests are indicated.
- Thyroid function test – if family history or sign and symptom suggestive of thyroid dysfunction.
- Wood light examination usually helps to localize the pigment to the epidermis or the dermis. In many cases, the pigment is found in both locations

Treatment

Melasma can be difficult to treat. The pigment of melasma develops gradually, and resolution is also gradual. Resistant cases or recurrences occur often and are certain if strict avoidance of sunlight is not rigidly heeded. All wavelengths of sunlight, including the visible spectrum, are capable of inducing melasma. The discoloration usually disappears spontaneously over a period of several months after giving birth or stopping the oral contraceptives or hormone replacement therapy. A course of hematinics (iron) will help women with anemia or nutritional deficiencies.

Treatments to hasten the fading of the discolored patches include:

- Hydroquinone (HQ) available in two strengths (2% and 4%), alone and in combination. It acts by inhibiting tyrosinase, an enzyme involved in the production of melanin.
- Tretinoin, an acid that increases skin cell (keratinocyte) turnover.
- Azelaic acid (20%), thought to decrease the activity of melanocytes. The primary adverse effect is skin irritation. No phototoxic or photoallergic reactions have been reported.
- Kojic acid, and ascorbic acid – other depigmenting agents
- Facial peel with alpha hydroxyacids (glycolic acid).
- Laser treatment.

  Cosmetic cover-ups can also be used to reduce the appearance of melasma.

Patient Education

- Strict sun avoidance is essential for resolution and to prevent recurrence. The use of broad-spectrum sunscreens with physical blockers, such as titanium dioxide and zinc dioxide is preferred over one with only chemical blockers.
- Patients should apply bleaching creams to areas of darkening only.
- Resolution with strict sun avoidance and topical depigmenting creams can take months; caution patients to expect slow but gradual lightening.

CRACKED FOOT

Cracked heel are a common foot problem which are a sign of lack of attention to foot care. For most people this is a nuisance and a cosmetic problem but when the fissures or cracks are deep, they are painful on standing; the skin can bleed and may become infected.

Some people tend to have a naturally dry skin that predisposes them to the cracks. The thickened dry skin (callus) around the heel that is more likely to crack is often due to mechanical factors that increase pressures in that area. Wearing open or thin soled shoes usually make the symptoms worse.

Factors that are involved in the cause of cracked heels include:

- Prolonged standing *especially on hard floor.*

- Being overweight *(this increases the pressure on the normal fat pad under the heel, causing it to expand sideways - if the skin is not supple and flexible, the pressures to 'crack' are high)*
- Open back on the shoes *(this allows the fat under the heel to expand sideways and increases the pressure to 'crack')*
- Some medical conditions predispose to a drying skin *(eg autonomic neuropathy in those with diabetes leads to less sweating; hypothyroidism- there is a reduction in sweating, leading to a dryness of the skin)*
- Skin diseases *(eg psoriasis and eczema)*

Advice for feet care -

- Avoid walking on bare feet.
- Removing the hard thick skin using pumice stone. This may need to be done on a regular basis. Never try to reduce the hard skin your self with a razor blade or a pair of scissors
- If cracks are very painful, strapping may be used to 'hold' the cracks together while they heal
- Wash the heels with warm water before going to bed and apply and massage in gently oil based moisturizing cream or emollient (petroleum jelly, coconut or sesame oil or a little ghee).
- Add rock salt to warm water and rest your feet in it.
- Change of footwear – wear footwear with closed back.
- A heel cup may be used to keep the fat pad from expanding sideways. This is worn in the shoe and can be very effective at prevention if used regularly.

  Regular maintenance may be the best way to prevent the problem.

STRETCH MARKS

Stretch marks are formed when the skin stretches at a rate that cannot be sustained by its elasticity. They may appear after rapid weight gain, spurts of growth and pregnancy. The development of breasts in adolescent girls and bulking up of muscles in weight lifters can also cause stretch marks. Women are more prone to stretch marks appearing on the breasts, lower abdomen, the buttocks and thighs.

They initially appear as red or purple lines of varying length or widths. Sometimes they are wrinkled and shiny. Gradually they fade to a shade lighter than the surrounding skin.

TREATMENT

1. The use of tretinoin has proven to be the most effective treatment to date -. Tretinoin when applied in high doses can cause a realignment of the collagen in the skin.

   To be effective, it must be applied in doses no less than 0.1% per day for a period of 12 weeks. The area becomes, very irritated dry and itchy. This reaction is important to the success of the treatment and must not be interfered by using moisturizing creams, or mild cortisone creams to ease discomfort.

   Stretch marks that have developed recently are more receptive to treatment with tretinoin than stretch marks which have been around for a while.
2. The next best treatment is to resurface the stretch marks with the carbon dioxide laser. This causes a reorganization of the collagen architecture in the skin.
3. In some cases the vascular removal laser may help to improve the look of stretch marks.
4. Another option is the use of injectable collagen. Zyplast collagen can be injected and molded into the depressed and thinned area of the stretch marks. The results are variable and not permanent and the amount of collagen that will be required to fill large areas of stretch marks would be very costly.
5. Linear surgical excision may help to select instances where a fine white scar would be preferable to unsightly stretch marks.
6. Opaque cosmetics, such as cover mark and derma blend may be used to camouflage visible stretch marks if they are particularly troublesome.

DARK UNDER EYE CIRCLE

These are generally caused by lack of sleep, fatigue, stress, dietary deficiency or associated with disorders like atopy. Proper sleep is vital for bright, shining eyes. Eight hours of sleep is a must.

Avoid extra strain on the eyes by reading only in good light and by making sure that you can see properly before undertaking work like sewing or writing.

The skin around the eye is very delicate. Adopt a daily care routine. Before going to sleep, clean the skin around the eyes with a moist cotton wool.

Almond helps to remove dark circles, and is an excellent "skin food".

Below are two simple home recipes to combat dark under eye circles:-

(A) Grate half cucumber, strain it and refrigerate. Dab a mixture of lemon juice, lanolin cream and cucumber juice around the eye for 10 minutes and then wipe off.

(B) Apply crushed mint around the eye carefully. This will take away the darkness around the eye.

ALLERGY TO ARTIFICIAL JEWELLERY

Allergy with artificial jewellery is common among women. They complaint of itching, redness and some times oozy lesions at the site of contact with the jewellery.

Most commonly it is the nickel content of the jewellery which is responsible for the allergy. Many individual become sensitized to nickel when their ears are pierced and made to wear nickel plated earrings. Nickel sensitivity will occur in 10% to 13% of patients if nickel plated earrings are inserted immediately after the ears are pierced. Dimethylglyoxime nickel spot test can detect nickel in artificial jewellery even in those made of nickel containing alloys.

Dermatitis is worse in summer as chloride radical in sweat is an important factor in dissolving the metallic nickel, permitting the soluble nickel salts to act.

Women develop skin lesions mostly at the site of contact with the jewellery. Sometimes they may develop skin eruption at distant sites like eyelids, elbow flexures, neck.

To prevent the development of allergy, gold or stainless steal earrings should be worn immediately following ear piercing.

Once a person develops allergy, she should not wear the jewellery any longer. If the allergic reaction is severe, or the reaction does not subside even after the exposure has ceased, then she should consult the dermatologist.

Sensitivity is likely to persist throughout life so if someone is keen on wearing favorite artificial jewellery, she may paint it with nail lacquer paint and wear for the shortest time possible.

SUN TANNING

Sun tanning describes a darkening of the skin (especially of fair-skinned individuals) in a natural physiological response stimulated by exposure to ultraviolet radiation from sunshine or from artificial sources such as a tanning bed.

The ultraviolet frequencies responsible for tanning are often divided into the UVA (315 to 400nm wavelength) and UVB (280 to 315nm wavelength) ranges. Firstly the UVA-radiation generates oxidative stress which in turn oxidises pre-existing melanin and it also causes release of preexisting melanin from the melanocytes.This leads to rapid darkening of already existing melanin.

While UVB causes increased production of melanin (melanogenesis). It is a reaction of the body to photodamage from UVB. Melanogenesis leads to delayed tanning. It first becomes visible about 72 hours after exposure and also lasts longer.

Measures to prevent tanning-

1. Avoid long sun exposures.
2. Use broad spectrum sunscreen with SPF factor of more than 15. Sunscreen should be hypoallergenic and noncomedogenic. Apply thick layer 15 to 30 minutes before exposure and one reapplication 15 to 30 minutes after the exposure begins.
3. Avoid sun between 10 a.m. and 2 p.m as sun rays strongest at this time.
4. Wear anti-UV sunglasses, hat with a brim, carry umbrellas.
5. Special sun protective clothing styling appropriate to full coverage of the skin can be worn. It is produced from a fabric (novel weave structure and denier -related to thread count per inch) rated for its level of ultraviolet (UV) protection

ENLARGED PORES

The over activity of the sebaceous glands usually results in skin with enlarged pores. Excessive oil secretion by the glands causes the pores to get clogged. The pores are thus stretched to accommodate the hardened sebum and lose their natural resilience. This excessive secretion of oil, might thicken the pores and mar the porcelain quality of skin, leaving the skin coarse.

CARE

(A) Use a medicated cleanser to reduce the surface oil and for deep pore cleansing

(B) The skin should be toned daily- it removes greasiness, closes pores, and refines the skin providing it a smooth clean texture. A skin tonic with a rose base is excellent. Keep some of it in a bowl in the refrigerator. Soak cotton wool pads and pat the skin briskly with it after a cleansing routine.

WRINKLES

Wrinkles are the thin, creased, and sagging skin that is especially noticeable on the face, neck, and hands.

Wind, heat and chemicals and the natural effects of aging cause a certain amount of wrinkling in everyone, but it is much worse in people who spend a lot of time in the sun.

Years of sun exposure cause the supporting structures of the skin, primarily the collagen and elastin, to weaken and break down. In addition, as a person ages, the sweat and oil glands of the skin become less numerous and smaller in size. This causes the skin to lose moisture and to dry out. Dry skin with weak collagen and elastin will sag, shrivel, and wrinkle.

In addition to sun exposure, smoking may contribute to the formation of wrinkles. Finally, it is believed that some wrinkling is predetermined genetically from one's parents.

Prevention- Onset of wrinkles and further progression of those already present can be prevented by following these tips:

1. Sun avoidance and sunscreen use- it is the most critical step in the prevention and treatment of wrinkles. Without these steps, even the more aggressive wrinkle treatments may be futile. Sun protection measures have been mentioned before.
2. Daily moisturizing creams- dry skin is more prone to wrinkling, so some recommend that daily moisturizing of skin should be done except in those with very oily skin.
3. Plenty of fresh fruits and vegetable intake.
4. Oral antioxidant – regular intake from younger age may prove beneficial

Treatment –

1. Medical – topical preparations containing tretinoin, alpha hydroxyl acids, chemical peels
2. Laser rejuvenation
3. Microdermabrasion
4. Dermal fillers for fixed wrinkles and botulinum toxin (Botox) injection for dynamic wrinkles.

CELLULITE

The bumpy, puckered and dimpled irregularities of fat collection which occurs over many women's buttocks, hips and thighs are called cellulite. These areas are often the first to attract fat and the last to lose it.

A mesh of collagen fibers hold the fat under the skin. The bumps, dimples and accompanying shadows of cellulite are simply the fat pushing out of the holes in the mesh.

In order to reduce cellulite,

- The amount of fat must be reduced.
- The supporting muscles must be toned up.
- The surroundings and intertwining protein mesh work needs to be altered.

Although cellulite is difficult to get rid off completely, a proper diet will reduce the fat, exercise will tone the underlying muscles and vigorous massaging will drown the protein mesh work and the fat stores, helping to improve the appearance of this condition.

Unfortunately there is no long term solution to cellulite. From a medical standpoint, topical aminophylline cream has been helpful for some people. The preparation is applied to the affected area twice a day to reduce cellulite in some people. Aminophylline cream is available only through medical prescription so do not go out searching in the local chemist shops.

The regular use of this cream in combination with the following suggestions should help to improve the look of the thighs and buttocks of women affected with cellulite:

- Maintaining lower fat stores, with a well balanced low fat diet.
- Avoid foods that encourage deep fluid retention, such as too much salt in the diet, and too many diet drinks.
- Regular hormonal balance, check-ups.

- Tone the muscles with daily buttocks, thigh and hip exercises, so that the fat cushion is sitting on a firm base. Exercise like vigorous walking, swimming and cycling are particularly helpful.
- Vigorous massaging the areas of cellulite for 10 min each day to break down the fibrous mesh and the larger fat globules.

If this fails to work and you are desperate, a combination of surgical liposuction to remove the fat from the bulges and fat transfer to place the fat in the dimples may even out the irregularities and permanently remove some of the fat stores.

DANDRUFF

Dandruff is a dry scaly condition of the skin on the scalp. It presents in two forms-

A) Pityriasis capitis- It is the milder kind consisting of white dry flakes over the scalp. The result is due to the rate at which the scalp sheds its dry skin cells, which in turn depends on the health and diet of the individual, stress too seems to be related.

Can be controlled by:-

(i) Paying more attention to scalp hygiene.
(ii) Consuming more fresh fruits in your diet.
(iii) Drinking plenty of water.
(iv) Rinsing the hair carefully after shampoo.
(v) Brushing gently to rid the hair of trapped cells.
(vi) Lightly massaging the scalp to dislodge the dandruff flakes.

If a simple routine like this does not work, consult a dermatologist on the use of anti-dandruff shampoo. Shampoos: Here are some ingredients in medicated shampoos that help control dandruff of the scalp-

- Tar
- Salicylic acid
- Zinc
- Selenium sulfide
- ketoconazole

(B) Seborrhoeic Dermatitis:- scalp has greasy, thick, yellowish scales.

This condition almost always needs medical care and attention by a dermatologist. Steroid based lotions and drugs to reduce yeast count need to be prescribed.

Hair Loss

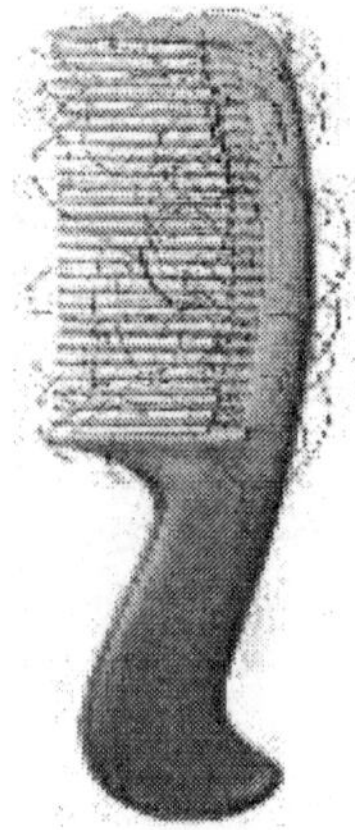

Nothing alarms women more than to be confronted with the problem of hair loss.

EXTERNAL FACTORS- The hair loss caused by these causes is not permanent as the roots have not been damaged. They will sprout new hair and it will grow back to its normal strength and thickness once the cause is removed and the hair thereafter treated with care.

(a) Styles that pull on hair for instance a ponytail, plait, or bun that's too tightly kept in place. Even frequently tugging on hair or nervously twisting may have the same outcome.

(b) Over-Zealous Brushing:- Especially with a brush made of plastic or metal.

(c) Traumatizing wet hair:- Using hair dryers or styling wet hair can break hair. Ideally towel-dry hair to get out the extra water, allow it to dry naturally.

(d) Avoid frequent use of heated, rollers and curling tongs for their can result in excessive loss of hair's natural oils and moisture, causing them to become brittle and break-prone.

(e) Subjecting hair to processes like bleaching dyeing or perming can lead to alter in molecular structure of hair.

(f) Use of harsh shampoos:- can make hair dry and brittle causing it to break off.

INTERNAL FACTORS

(a) Hormonal factors – androgen sensitivity leads to frontotemporal baldness in males and female pattern hair loss in some females, thyroid disorders.

(b) Nutritional deficiency of iron, proteins, minerals in diet produce hair fall.
(c) Connective tissue diseases.
(d) Stress-
(e) Drugs- chemotherapeutic agents, retinoids

TIPS ON MANAGING HAIR LOSS

Following measures may be taken and if hair fall continues, then one should contact a dermatologist for evaluation and investigation for the cause of excessive hair fall.

- Brushing of hair should be gentle. Use a brush with natural bristles to avoid tearing the hair. You can also use a nylon brush with smooth rounded bristles.
- Avoid excessive brushing, for it might pull the hair, causing breakage.
- Avoid using harsh shampoos, which might again leave the hair dry and brittle.
- Avoid vigorous scalp massage, for it will lead to further hair loss.
- Choose products formulated for one's hair type.

If sudden, extensive hair loss occurs, medical attention should be sought immediately

Greying of hair

The hair has a tendency to lose its natural colour with advancing age and turn grey, but premature greying is a morbid condition and it makes even the young look older. Pigment cells that are present at the base of the hair follicle stop producing pigment, which leads to lose of original hair colour and inturn graying of hairs. Melanocytes are the cells that produce melanin, which is responsible for the colour of the body and hair. With aging, melanocytes lose their ability in producing pigments, which leads to greying. Grey hair is usually associated with ageing, but this is not always the case.

Many factors play role in it-

1. Heredity – Genetics plays a very significant role.
2. Malnutrition - A faulty diet lacking in B vitamins, iron, copper, and iodine in the daily diet is said to be a contributory factor.
3. Physical or mental stress

4. Constant mental worrying.
5. Sever illness too can stop or affect the production of melanin.
6. Washing hair in hot water, drying hair using an electric dryer.

Home Remedies

The use of Indian gooseberry 'amla' is the foremost among the home remedies found beneficial in the prevention and treatment of premature greying of hair. This is a valuable hair tonic for enriching hair growth and hair pigmentation.

Amaranth is another effective home remedy for hair disorders. Application of the fresh juice of the leaves of this vegetable helps the hair to retain its black colour and prevents it from premature greying.

Liberal intake of curry leaves is considered beneficial in preventing premature greying of hair.

The butter made from cow's milk has the property of preventing premature greying of hair. A small roll may be taken internally and a little quantity may be massaged into the hair roots twice a week.

Proper grooming is very important to keep the hair texture, growth, shin and luster in a good condition. Therefore use a shampoo and conditioner that suits your hair type. Choose products that are gentle, preferably without any harsh detergent like sodium lauryl sulfate.

Nourishment

Your hair needs the following nourishment:

(a) **Vitamin A** - It is necessary for promoting a healthy scalp and gives body and glow to your hair. Include dark green vegetables and orange and yellow fruits and vegetables in your diet.

(b) **Vitamin B** - It regulates the secretion of oil, keeps hair healthy & moisturized. Eat more of fresh green leafy vegetables, tomatoes, cauliflower, cereals, liver kidney, yogurt, bananas and green vegetables.

(c) **Minerals** - Zinc, iron & copper promote healthy hair. Food sources: zinc - red meat, chicken & green vegetables; iron - beef, dried apricots, red meat, parsley, eggs, wheat & sunflower seeds; copper - seafood, egg yolk & whole grains.

(d) **Proteins** - consuming more of protein gives your hair natural shine and good texture. Include more of sprouted whole grains, cereals, meat and soy in your diet.

The vitamins considered useful in guarding against premature greying of hair are pantothenic acid, para-aminobenzoic acid (PABA), inositol. The minimum daily requirement of these vitamins appears to be 10 mg of pantothenic acid, 100 mg of para-aminobenzoic acid, and 2 gm of inositol. To obtain satisfactory results, all three of these vitamins belonging to the B group should be supplied at one time, preferably in a form which supplies all the B vitamins, such as yeast and liver. The three anti-greying-hair vitamins can also be produced in the intestinal tract by bacteria.Thus, taking a sufficient quantity of yoghurt daily and a tablespoonful of yeast before each meal is an excellent remedy for the prevention and treatment of premature greying of hair.

Juice of carrot, lettuce, capsicum and fresh alfalfa remove copper deficiency, this is good remedy for gray hair and hair loss.

Massage of the scalp with almond oil is recommended

Devitalising foods such as white flour, refined sugar and all products made from them, soft drinks, pastries, jams and jellies should be avoided. These foods take away energy, cause wrinkles, unattractive skin, grey hair, and premature old age.

Daily gentle massage your scalp and hair with your fingertips; it helps maintain proper blood circulation in the scalp.

Take a cup of strong black tea (without milk), and to this add a tablespoon of salt. When cold, strain the tea and massage it on the roots. Leave it on for an hour, and then rinse with cold water. Do not shampoo it.

Massage your hairs with coconut oil and lemon everyday for at least 15 minutes.

Dyeing

Dyeing is one of the most common ways of treating grey hair. Chemical dyes sold in the markets aid in colouring your hair. Though it is the most opted way, some people do not prefer it due to the reaction of its chemical properties on the hair and scalp.

Henna colouring

Henna colouring is one of the natural and traditional ways of treating grey hair. Henna cools the body as well as renders softness apart from colouring the hair.

Do's and don'ts of healthy hair –

- Choose brushes and combs with widely spaced and smooth tipped bristles and teeth to avoid the risk of splitting hairs and scratching the scalp.
- Wash combs and brushes in shampoo or soap at least once a week.
- Always rinse your hair thoroughly.
- Use a conditioner to smooth the outer surface of the hair, which is roughened by washing.
- Apply extra conditioner when using a hairdryer, rollers, or tongs.
- Always try a temporary rinse first, before you risk using permanent color.
- Go to a professional colorist for permanent dyeing or bleaching.
- Don't over brush your hair, for it may increase the greasiness of oily hair and break the ends of dry hair.
- Don't tangle the hair while washing it.
- Don't give dry hair two applications of shampoo.
- Don't rub hair too vigorously when drying, it may break and tangle the hair.
- Don't have a permanent bleach if all you really need are "highlights".
- Don't apply a permanent color until you have tested the solution on your skin for 36 hours to check for any adverse reactions.
- By using very mild shampoos and good quality conditioners.
- By having them trimmed regularly.
- By going in for once-weekly hot oil treatment. Use warm olive or almond oil and massage it carefully into the scalp and hair.
- Leave the oil on overnight, if possible, by covering the hair with a plastic bath cap and a toweling turban. Wash the oil off the next day by applying diluted shampoo directly to the scalp before applying water.

NAILS

Brittle nails

Brittle nails is a condition where the nails are fragile and break frequently. Dry and brittle nails often worsen in low humidity and in the winter (dry heat). **Brittle nails** can occur otherwise but they can also be an indication of several other medical conditions including nutritional disorder, iron deficiency anemia, hypothyroidism and infections.

Every day, fingernails put in hard labor – tapping on desktops, opening envelops, digging in the garden, or scratching off the peel on instant win lottery cards. Fingernails are incredibly strong and can usually withstand all the abuse. After about age thirty, however, people's nails get weaker and more brittle. This can cause them to break or splinter, or simply look a little more ragged than they used to.

Some tips for healthy nails-

1. Wearing gloves when performing household chores that involve getting the hands wet is very helpful in preventing brittle nails. Cotton lined rubber gloves can be purchased in stores.
2. Apply lotions containing alpha-hydroxy acids or lanolin containing lotions to the nails after first soaking nails in water for 5 minutes.
3. Avoid harsh chemicals such as detergents, cleaning fluids and nail polish removers (the acetone containing removers are somewhat worse than acetone free).
4. Be gentle to you nails. Shape and file the nails with a very fine file and round the tips in a gentle curve.
5. Avoid metal instruments on the nail surface to push back the cuticle.
6. Daily filing of snags or irregularities helps to prevent further breakage or splitting.
7. Do not use poor quality nail paint and nail polishes with nylon fibers in them may add strength to the nails.
8. Biotin (a vitamin) taken by mouth is beneficial in some people. Lentils and peanuts, along with cauliflower, are rich sources of biotin.
9. Fish- salmon, mackerel, and other cold – water fish contain fatty acids, which the body uses to strengthen the nails.
10. Moisturize nails with little bit of petroleum jelly once or twice a day; nails naturally get hard and brittle whenever they dry out.

11. Avoid frequent soaking and drying of nails as nails expand when they absorb water, then contract when then dry. The more this cycle is repeated, the weaker the nails become.
12. **Treat them with respect – though** fingernails are tough shouldn't expect them to do double-duty as tools. Scissors, screwdrivers, staple removers, and tweezers were all invented for a reason.
13. **Cover them up-** wear gloves whenever you're putting your hands to work in rough environments – in a sink full of hot, soapy water, for example, or in a mound of garden soils
14. **Keep them trimmed-** Long nails are more fragile and break more easily than short ones.

PARONYCHIA

Paronychia is a soft tissue infection around a fingernail. Paronychia occurs in 2 forms: acute and chronic. The etiology, infectious agent, and treatment are usually different for each form, and the 2 forms are often considered separate entities.

Paronychia, whether acute or chronic, results from a breakdown of the protective barrier between the nail and the nail fold. This facilitates entry of organisms into the moist nail crevice resulting in the bacterial or fungal (yeast or mold) colonization of the area.

Paronychia is the most commonly encountered hand infection. Susceptible people include those whose occupations require them to have their hands in prolonged contact with water; include bartenders, florists, bakers, and homemakers.

It may occur in patients of all ages and women are affected more than men.

• Acute paronychia

- The presenting complaints are pain, tenderness, and swelling in one of the lateral folds of the nail.
- Patients with acute paronychia often give history of minor trauma to the fingertip or nail manipulation, intentional or not. This breaks down the physical barrier between the nail fold and the nail plate; this disruption allows the infiltration of infectious organisms most commonly staphylococcus aureus.

- In more advanced cases, pus may collect under the skin of the lateral fold.
  - Chronic paronychia
- Chronic paronychia is primarily caused by the yeast fungus *Candida albicans*.
- Generally, patients complain of symptoms lasting 6 weeks or longer.
- Recurrent episodes of inflammation, pain, and swelling of nailfold.
- Nail plates become thickened and discolored, with pronounced transverse ridges.
- Swollen, erythematous, and tender nail folds without fluctuance are characteristic of chronic paronychia.
- Chronic paronychia most often occurs in persons whose hands are repeatedly exposed to moist environments or in those who have prolonged and repeated contact with irritants such as mild acids, mild alkalis, or other chemicals. People who are most susceptible include housekeepers, dishwashers, bartenders, and swimmers.

Medical Care

The treatment of choice depends on the extent of the infection.

Acute paronychia

If diagnosed early, without obvious abscess formation, it can be treated with medicine salon. If an abscess has developed, incision and drainage must be performed.

- Warm water soaks of the affected finger 3-4 times per day until symptoms resolve.
- Oral antibiotics with gram-positive coverage against *S aureus,* such as amoxicillin and clavulanic acid (Augmentin) or clindamycin (Cleocin),
- If the paronychia does not resolve or if it progresses to an abscess, it should be drained promptly.

Chronic paronychia

- Avoidance of inciting factors such as exposure to moist environments or skin irritants.

- Keep hands clean and dry. Treatment is unlikely to be successful if their exposure to moist or wet environment is not changed.
- Any manipulation of the nail, or trauma such as manicuring, finger sucking, or attempting to incise and drain the lesion, should be avoided as this can lead to secondary bacterial infections.
- Mild cases of chronic paronychia may be treated with warm soaks.
- The initial medical treatment consists of the application of topical antifungal agents (miconazole). Oral ketoconazole or fluconazole may be added in more severe cases.
- Patients with diabetes and those who are immunocompromised need more aggressive treatment because the response to therapy is slower in these patients.

Suggested further reading

1. A Woman's Skin by David M., M.D. Stoll
2. Skin Care: Beyond the Basics by Mark Lees
3. The Wrinkle Cure By Nicholas Perricone, MD
   Pure skin - Organic Beauty Basics by Barbara Close

36

Sleep Problems in Women

Siddalingaiah H S and Amarjeet Singh

Sleep is one of the most elemental human needs and accounts for one third of human life. Most adults sleep 7 to 8 hours per night although the timing, duration, and internal structure of sleep vary among healthy individuals and as a function of age. Adults of intermediate age tend to have one consolidated sleep episode per day. Good sleep has been listed as essential for maintaining good health. It has been documented that poor sleep contributes to ill health. Epidemiologic studies show that abnormal sleep patterns predict lower life expectancy, cardiovascular disease risk, predisposition to prostatic cancer, breast cancer, etc.

Sleep disorders are encountered in all age groups and all societies and sections. The prevalence varies in different settings starting from 5-10 % in general population.

All over the world sleep problems in women are common in perimenopausal age group affecting more than 38% of them. The menopausal transition, independent of other potential explanatory factors, is associated with self-reported sleep difficulty.[1]

Both menopause related as well as unrelated factors play a role in the causation of sleep problems in women. [5]

There are different types of sleep problems,

1. Insomnia (sleep problem at night with excessive daytime sleepiness)

Insomnia is the most common sleep problem. Women are more likely than men to report insomnia. In fact, according to the 2002 NSF Sleep in America poll, more women than men experience symptoms of insomnia at least a few nights a week (63% vs. 54%) and they are more likely to have daytime sleepiness. Sometimes, women begin to have sleepless nights associated with menstruation, pregnancy or menopause and find it difficult to break poor sleep habits.[2, 6]

2. Sleep Apnea (sleep time breathing problem)
Sleep apnea is a serious sleep disorder that is characterized by snoring, interrupted breathing during sleep and excessive daytime sleepiness. An estimated 18 million Americans have sleep apnea including one in four women over 65. While apnea is more common in men, it increases in women after age 50. Because being overweight is a risk factor for sleep apnea, the increase in abdominal fat during menopause may be one reason menopausal women are 3.5 times as likely to get this sleep disorder. Some attribute the prevalence to hormonal changes such as the decrease in progesterone.[2, 6]
3. Restless Legs Syndrome (RLS) and Periodic Limb Movement Disorder (PLMD)
RLS is a neurological movement disorder that affects as many as 12 million Americans.. Because the unpleasant feelings occur at rest and are relieved by movement, RLS sufferers have difficulty sleeping. In the NSF 2002 *Sleep in America* poll, 18% of the female adult population reported RLS symptoms a few nights a week or more.[2a, 2b]

Causative factors for sleep problems:

1. Overweight[6]
2. Menopausal hormonal changes
3. Depression[6]
4. Poor sleep hygiene practices, e.g. Not observing a regular time for going to bed
5. Working women; flotation shift works
6. Smoking, caffeine, alcohol
7. Family conflicts
8. Medical problems; chronic illnesses
9. Low backache, bone thinning (osteoporosis)
10. Acid reflux disease (acidity/gas/indigestion)

11. Incontinence (urine leakage).[3, 2b]

Prevention and management of sleep problems:

It should be realized that, essentially much of the sleep problems can be tackled without using any medicine as sleep is a part of our daily routine. Try to manage it without using medicine. You are capable of sound sleep without any artificial assistance majority of the times. Good sleep habits can help you get a good night's sleep. Here are some tips:

- Try to go to bed at the same time every night and get up at the same time every morning. Try not to take naps during the day because naps may make you less sleepy at night.
- Try to avoid caffeine, nicotine, and alcohol late in the day. Caffeine and nicotine are stimulants and can keep you from falling asleep. Alcohol can make you wake up later in the night.
- Get regular exercise.
- But try not to exercise close to bedtime because it may stimulate you and make it hard to fall asleep. Experts suggest not exercising for 3 hours before the time you go to sleep.
- Don't eat a big meal late in the night. There should be a gap between your dinner and bedtime.
- Make your sleeping place comfortable. Be sure that it is dark, quiet, and not too warm or too cold. If light is a problem, try a sleeping mask. If noise is a problem, try earplugs or a fan to cover up the sounds.
- Create a routine to help you relax and wind down before sleep, such as reading a book or taking a bath. Watching the news just before bed may keep some people awake, especially if the news is upsetting.
- Try not to use your bed for anything other than sleeping and sex.
- If you can't fall asleep and don't feel sleepy, get up and do something else until you feel sleepy. Just make sure that you don't do anything stimulating.
- If you have trouble lying awake worrying about things, try making a to-do list before you go to bed. This may help you to "let go" of those worries overnight.[2a,2b]

Time to consult a doctor:

Insomnia problem is said to be persisting if in spite of above mentioned non medical methods fail to reduce daytime sleepiness, fatigue, concentration difficulties, etc. after complying with them for more 3 weeks.

- If insomnia persists, and lifestyle, behavioral or diet changes do not help, a doctor may prescribe a sleep-promoting medication (hypnotic).
- In some instances, there may be an underlying and treatable cause, such as depression (women are twice as likely to report depression as men), stress, anxiety, reflux, bladder problems or pain.
- Doctors may prescribe antidepressants or anti-anxiety drugs, medications for heartburn, incontinence or pain and/or hypnotic medications to improve sleep.[2a,4]

However, there is enough evidence to suggest that non-medical methods are to be preferred over medical methods since use of hypnotics, sedatives, sleep pills have side effects which include loss of memory for the events that occur after the drug is administered, hangover effect on the next morning, drowsiness, impaired performance and judgement. Some are not suitable for people with asthma, respiratory problems; they can cause addiction; not to be given in pregnancy and to breast feeding mothers as they are dangerous for the fetus and the baby. They can also cause changes in appetite, changes in urination, constipation, lethargy, vertigo, visual disturbances.[7] Thus, sleep inducing drugs have many problems.

In one study, there was a relationship between suicide rates among various groups of people and total sales of these drugs in that population area.[8]

In another study among elderly people there was an increased suicide rate among those using benzodiazepine and other hypnotics like flunitrazepam and nitrazepam. The terminal cause of death was drowning, often in the victim's own bathtub, in three-quarters of them. The annual fatality ratios even for the newer benzodiazepine-like hypnotics zopiclone and zolpidem appear to be on the rise. Hence they should be prescribed with caution for this age group.[9]

Any person who uses sleep inducing drugs is likely to have a stock of such medicine at home and this can be a facilitating factor for suicide.

References

1. Kravitz, Howard M.; Ganz, Patricia A.; Bromberger, Joyce; Powell, Lynda H.; Sutton-Tyrrell, Kim; Meyer, Peter M. Sleep difficulty in women at midlife: a community survey of sleep and the menopausal transition. Menopause 2003; 10:19-28.

2a. http://www.womenshealthzone.net/sleep-disorders/overview/prevention

2b. http://www.sleepeducation.com/Topic, from American Academy of Sleep Medicine

3. Wikipedia, the free encyclopedia by Wikimedia Foundation, Inc., http://en.wikipedia.org/wiki/Sleep. http://en.wikipedia.org/wiki/Insomnia.

4. Suzanne Barston, Heather Larson, Gina Kemp, M.A., and Robert Segal, M.A. Helpguide: A project of the Rotary Club of Santa Monica and WISE & Healthy Aging. http://www.helpguide.org/life/sleep_disorders.htm.

5. Young T, Rabago D, Zgierska A, Austin D, Laurel F. Objective and subjective sleep quality in premenopausal, perimenopausal, and postmenopausal women in the Wisconsin Sleep Cohort Study. Sleep. 2003 Sep; 26:667-72.

6. Basta M, Lin HM, Pejovic S, Sarrigiannidis A, Bixler E, Vgontzas AN. Lack of regular exercise, depression, and degree of apnea are predictors of excessive daytime sleepiness in patients with sleep apnea: sex differences. J Clin Sleep Med. 2008 Feb 15; 4:19-25.

7. Laurence L. Brunton, Keith L. Parker, Iain L. O. Buxton, and Donald K. Blumenthal. Goodman & Gilman's The Pharmacological Basis of Therapeutics, 11th Edition. McGraw-Hill Companies publications.

8. Sundquist J, Ekedahl A, Johansson S. Sales of tranquillizers, hypnotics/sedatives and antidepressants and their relationship with underprivileged area score and mortality and suicide rates. European journal of clinical pharmacology. 1996 Oct 51; 2:105-109.

9. Carlsten A, Waern M, Holmgren P, Allebeck P. The role of benzodiazepines in elderly suicides. Scand J Public Health. 2003; 31(3):224-8.

37

Spiritual Health of Women

NK Goel, MK Sharma and Abhiruchi Galhotra

INTRODUCTION

Over the last several decades, the topic of spirituality has come to forefront of public and professional consciousness. Spirituality encompasses all aspects of being human and is a means of experiencing life. Spirituality is a multidimensional phenomenon that transcends gender, race, colour and national origin. It is individualistic and involves a series of steps or cycles that occur in no particular order or timeframe throughout the life of an individual.

Defying development of a standard definition, spirituality remains a highly subjective, personal and individualist concept.

The term "Spirituality" is derived from the Latin Spiritus meaning breath. It is also related to Greek 'pnenma' or breath, which refers to the vital spirit or soul. Spirituality refers to the "human propensity to find meaning in life through self-transcendence; it is evident in a sense of relatedness to… something greater than the self; it may or may not include formal religious participation." A strong sense of Spirituality may be associated with a meaningful relationship with the Divine, a deep sense of belonging to a greater whole or of participating in the universe, and healing experiences.

A contemporary Western theologian, Paul Tillich, has written about religion and spirituality. Rejecting a theist definition, he maintained that religion was "that which is ultimate, infinite, unconditional" in one's life and "the state of being grasped by an ultimate concern. Religious concerns involve serious issues such as the meaning of life; concerns that are more finite or less important are not religious. Religious beliefs are significant guiding forces in people's decisions and actions; religious practices are those that one regards as having ultimate meaning. Tillich's concept of religion as ultimate is compatible with feminist, Spiritual traditions and is not characterized by androcentrism or an anthropomorphized male deity. Tillich's concept of the Ultimate is relevant to, and consistent with assumptions in women's Spirituality (Dr. Kelly Denton-Borhaug, Stanford University, personal communication, February 1999). Despite the fact that the spirituality is not well defined, its role in comprehension of health and health care is emerging as a valuable and important concept. More than half the doctors now realise that it is extremely important.

CHARACTERISTICS OF SPIRITUAL HEALTH

Although, there is no way to actually measure spiritual health, the state of spiritual health can be defined as consisting of following characteristics:-

1. Sense of inner peace
2. Ability to find comfort and/or strength in one's spiritual beliefs and values.
3. Belief in one's own worth and goodness
4. Belief in divine or perpetual goodness
5. Ability to receive and offer love and care.
6. Strong connection to people
7. Sense of purpose in world.
8. Ability to forgive self and others
9. Hopefulness in future
10. Sense of some control over one's own life.

WOMEN AND HEALTH

Women make incredible contributions to society as parents, workers, and leaders in spirituality and health care.[3] Women's health is important not only to women but also to their families, their communities and the world as a whole. The very progress of civilization depends on the unconstrained participation of women in all aspects of social life. Participation requires that women and girls be assisted and encouraged to develop all of their capacities and that they maintain their ongoing physical, emotional and spiritual health essentials to contribute as equal partners with men to the advancement of civilization. Women play fundamental roles in the education of children and in promoting the health of family both at home, and through organizations that promote, protect the health and well being of the community. Healthy families and communities cannot be achieved without careful attention to creating conditions conducive to sustaining healthy girls and women as well.

To clarify, the term health is used here to encompass both illness and well-being. Illness and well-being are separate concepts: each exists on a separate continuum. The absence of illness does not indicate the presence of health. Illness may be thought of as a human response to discomfort and disease. Well-being may be characterized by positive states or functioning in multiple dimensions (i.e physically, cognitively, emotionally, psychologically, socially and spiritually). Consistent with conceptualizations of well-being, women's health practice involves building "supporting environments in which women can thrive rather than merely survive".

For improving the health of women/girls- awareness of the rights of women and girls should be raised, raising the discussion of issues to the level of principle and applying them at the local, national and global levels. When women's experiences with stressful events such as harassment, violence or abuse are listened to and responded to by groups or communities, women's health is said to be improving. It is through relationships with others that many women learn who they are and what is of ultimate importance. Relationships are central to women's psychological development and are integral to women's empowerment and to women's social roles. Having warm, caring relationships with others is as important as the psychological well being and physical health of women.

Increasingly, women have been co-participating in their health care experiences both outside and inside the health care system. In women's **groups** focused on health, women are teaching themselves about self – identified issues (self defense, healthy eating and relationships). Women are encouraged to participate in the assessment of their own bodies (taking their own BP or weight etc.).

EMPOWERING WOMEN REGARDING HEALTH

Through interactions, women can experience mutual engagement, empathy, and empowerment. Having warm, caring relationships with others is important for psychological well-being and physical heath. Having positive relationships with a Divine presence also is associated with general well-being (e.g., happiness in life and marriage).

De-constructing traditional androcentric health systems and reconstructing definitions of good health care for women have occurred in several ways. Leaders in the women's health movement have demonstrated how women can take health care into their own hands. They have challenged the myth of medical control and the role of passive patients. In health care settings, they have reconstructed more egalitarian roles and relationships between practitioners and clients. They have set new expectations for continuity of care with clinicians and demand for more comprehensive services offered, including complementary and alternative therapies. To the degree that health care systems are now responding to women's health care demand more fully, Women's voices are being heard.

Tillich believed that spiritual well-being can emerge from struggling with, and healing from, threats to one's physical health. Spiritual experiences of self- transcendence have been correlated inversely with depression and mental distress.

Intrinsic spirituality is the belief that God or a Higher Power exists, that one feels close to such a God, and that this God dwells within. Intrinsic spirituality has been associated positively with life satisfaction and health promoting attitudes, and negatively with symptoms. Spirituality that was chosen actively (i.e. through identification) rather than passively accepted (i.e. through introspection) was associated with positive psychological states. Thus, what may be important to health is how one is religious, rather than whether one is religious.

Although clinicians and clergy may be catalysts for empowerment, they cannot empower women: individual women ultimately empower themselves. The outcomes of spiritual and health processes often involve transformation of individual women (e.g. their identity, roles, or value of selves).

In both perspectives, leaders are changing traditional androcentric, paternalistic systems that have affected women's bodies, minds, and spirits negatively. In both perspectives, leaders are challenging traditions and reconstructing new norms. Both clergy and community health practitioners are working to change and improve women's lives collectively and to build systems that foster women's growth.

WOMEN'S SPIRITUALITY AND HEALTH

Clergy and health practitioners can encourage and support integration and healing among women in several ways. Clergy and practitioners can encourage quieting- being still and present. This is the approach of mindfulness – to be aware of the present most fully, forgetting past events and letting go of future hopes. Mindfulness practices have been associated with reduction in physical and psychological symptoms

Clergy and clinicians can promote women's listening within. Listening within can occur when women tune out the noise of the world and let go of daily hassles. Reflection may aid in the identification of what is of Ultimate importance and may be stimulated by silent contemplation, journal writing, meditation, or prayer. After such reflection, women may have identified priorities more clearly and be able to better act on them.

Those who are facilitators of women's spirituality and women's health can invite women to engage in self-nurturing activities and to legitimize these activities. Such nurturing activities are most often self-identified, but may include taking a warm bath, having a massage, listening to music, or being in nature. A nurse researcher has shown that taking time for restorative activities such as watching a sunset or gardening can increase one's cognitive abilities to cope with a major illness. Women who have stress-related conditions may experience reduced psychological distress and better functioning after taking time for themselves.

Clinicians and clergy can create and support opportunities for women's sharing and validating experiences in their bodies, minds, spirits, and lives. Clinicians and clergy can create sacred spaces in which women can connect with themselves and each other, develop inner strengths, facilitate empowerment, and experience personal transformation and healing.

Clinicians and clergy may facilitate small groups and communities to create environments for empowerment and transformation. For example, groups designed for women who are coping with a particular chronic illness or stressor can provide opportunities for such women to learn to cope better with health threats or to deal more effectively with stressful life events. In such groups, women may claim their beliefs more strongly and speak their minds more clearly. Through interactions with other in such groups, sharing and validation of women's reflections and resources can occur, as well as experience of empowerment, healing and transformation.

In communities or larger groups, rituals may include thematic readings, collective reflection, meditation, singing, dancing, discussion, and participatory exercise. Rituals can honor, on individual and collective levels, the meaningful transformations in women's development (eg. menarche, menopause, coming out, or freedom from addiction). In such rituals, it is not unusual for women to experience a sense of empowerment.

WOMEN AND SPIRITUAL HEALTH

Spirituality is an integral part of the health, healing and well being of every individual. It is expressed and experienced through interconnectedness with Nature, the earth, the environment, the cosmos and the other people. Spirituality is intertwined with every aspect of life. It provides purpose, meaning, strength and guidance in shaping the journey of life.[1] Women's health involves the interplay of social, individual and biological factors and is experienced within physical, emotional, intellectual, social and spiritual dimensions. Studies generally support the hypothesis that spirituality is correlated with favorable health care outcomes.

Men and women have different skills. Now-a-days, female managers score over men with several qualities like team work, decision making ability, collaboration, patience, commitment, devotion, etc which are inherent in women. Women are superior to men in spirituality. They have subtler senses; they are more sensitive, compassionate and loving, more mystic and get easily enlightened. It is the social, cultural and religious circumstances which make them feel suppressed. To overcome this, women need to get right knowledge about themselves and their potential. They have to really know about their body, their mind, their relationship and their spiritual self.

As you work upon gaining this knowledge, you can gain confidence, find right relationships, love others and yourself, come out of conditions and fear. The fact is that women don't love themselves. Every woman feels oneself not good enough. Except for God only women can create that is to give birth. It requires compassion and patience. This is women's real skill and is certainly women's potent power. Being spiritual means gaining access to the higher energy, connecting to God and the guider within. When your life is led by Him, He will do everything for you. Women are spiritual being. Develop your spirituality. Spirituality is how you relate with everything. It is a way of life. It is neither an idea nor a religion nor a 'do this and not do that'.

SPIRITUAL HEALTH AND RELIGION

Religiosity, a concept related with spirituality refers to religious attendance, practice or activity. Religiosity influences the response to signs and symptoms of illness through rituals associated with diseases prevention and health protection. Social, moral and dietary prescriptions that promote health and communal religious activities that increase social support are among the effects of religious involvement.

Religion is usually recognized as the practical expression of spirituality. Religion is derived from Latin world 'Religare' - which means to bind together. Mathews & Clark propose the following distinctions both religion and spirituality:

(a) Religion focuses on establishing community, while spirituality emphasises individual growth.
(b) Religion is easier to identify and objectively measure than spirituality.
(c) Religion is more formal in worship, more authoritarian in its directions, more orthodox and systematic in doctrine and has more formally prescribed and proscribed behaviour than spirituality.

(d) While religion is more behaviour based and focused on outward, observable practices, spritiuality is more emotion based and focused on inner experiences

(e) While religion is particular, segregating one group from another, spirituality is more universal, emphasizing community and unity with others.

(f) Individuals with life threatening or chronic health conditions can benefit greatly from spirituality and religious practices.

(g) Religious beliefs had a positive impact on spiritual well being in women with breast carcinoma.

(h) Spirituality is believed to play a crucial role in an individual's recovery from acute illness and surgery.

(i) Spirituality seems to improve resistance, well being and ability to cope with difficult life events in those people with HIV/AIDS.

(j) Religious activities enhance people's ability to cope with many chronic illnesses i.e. cystic fibrosis, DM, CRF etc.

(k) Many terminally ill individuals derive great strength and hope from their religious and spiritual beliefs.

Many people find spirituality through religion or through a personal relationship with the divine. Study of the world's religions reveals that each religion attempts to answer mankind's spiritual questions and that each have developed a specific set of beliefs, teachings and practices. A person's experience with religious organizations may range from extremely positive to extremely negative.

A growing body of research focuses specifically on the relationship between spirituality and health among women of color. Rojas postulated that high levels of spiritual well-being and frequent church attendance allow low-income Hispanic women to cope with the stresses of poverty and remain essentially healthy. An ethnographic study of Hispanic women demonstrated an emphasis on the importance of spirituality and the integration of the spiritual dimension as important to healthy living.

A significant positive correlation was shown between religious well-being and the variables of social support and hope in study of elderly women, while spirituality was cited as a facilitator of mental well being. Religion and spirituality are often associated with the ability to cope with adverse health experiences. For example, African American and Puerto Rican women living with HIV/AIDS identified spirituality as an important dimension of healthy living and potential growth, emphasizing the influence of prayer, television, ministries, and Bible reading.

HEALTH AND PRAYER

Prayer is the most common form of spiritual ritual and is practiced by religious as well as non-religious individuals throughout the world. There are numerous studies that demonstrate a significant correlation between spirituality and healing and prayer and healing. It is reported that 82% of Americans believe in the healing power of personal prayers.

TECHNIQUES FOR PRAYING:-

- Relaxation, quieting and breath awareness
- Attention training and focusing
- Imaging and visualization
- Intentionality
- Movement such as dancing, walking etc
- Inspirational or sacred readings
- Anointing with oil
- Singing
- Meditation
- Music
- Chanting

TYPES OF PRAYERS

1. Petitioner prayer: -Involves asking a Higher Power to respond to a specific request
2. Intercessory Prayer:- "Distant Prayer" petitioner prayer on behalf of others
3. Adoration Prayer:- Involves praising & glorifying a higher power
4. Ritual Prayer: involves the repetition if prayers created by another and involves using spiritual readings, repetition, rosary or a prayer book.
5. Meditative or contemplative prayer: Involves opening of the mind & heart to a higher power that transcends words or thoughts.

6. Colloquial prayer: Involves communicating with the divine in an informal, honest and self revealing manner as if talking to a friend.

MEDITATION:

It is a ritual and a process to spiritual transformation. It is a learned skill. It originated in ancient India about 3000 yrs ago and exists in major religious and many secular organizations.

It is a learned skill and provides with many physiological benefits, such as stress reduction, decreased adrenaline flow, decreased BMR, decreased HR, relaxation and decreased pain. Also, it may lead to new insights about life issues, increased creativity, inspiration, greater compassion for others etc.

During meditation, a person's attention and concentration are intentionally trained. All meditative techniques involve conscious breathing and a focus on what is happening in each present moment until the mind becomes empty of thoughts, judgments and past and future concerns. To enter into meditative state, the following methods may be helpful:-

(a) Breathing techniques
(b) Meditating with sound – mantras, chanting, drums, audiotapes
(c) Meditating with visualization – picturing a sacred place, focusing on an external object. Visualizing sacred symbols.

EMPIRICISM:

Though many people assert that there is substantial empirical support for the idea that religious activities promote health & are also associated with reduced mortality, yet, for several reasons, such epidemiologic studies do not provide justification for physicians to encourage patients to attend religious services or to engage in other religious activities. First, the strongest evidence of an effect of religion on health comes from studies of only church attendance, though other religious activities might also be associated.Second, diversity in style and content of prayer are not considered.Third, epidemiologic studies reflect only associations at the population level. It must be confirmed by rigorous clinical trials, but since any effects on health are likely to differ according to whether patients attended religious services on their own or because of a physician's recommendations, such a trial would be problematic and difficult to conduct.

Even in the absence of supporting evidence, it would still be permissible for physicians to recommend that patients engage in religious activities because such activities provide comfort. The authors state, "The primary task of the physician is **'to cure sometimes, to relieve often, and to comfort always"**. It is certainly true that for many patients, religion provides comfort in times of difficulty.

Physicians have considerable influence, which presumably derives from their medical expertise, and patients often regard their recommendations as authoritative. For example, the recommendations that a patient with pneumonia takes antibiotics and restricts his or her activity are likely to be followed because the patient accepts the physician's authority. The same influence is exerted when a physician inquires about or recommends religious activities. Physicians and patients alike are on dangerous ground if they believe that advice about religious matters has the same medical support as a recommendation for antibiotic treatment. Such assumptions can have a coercive effect, and they raise ethical questions about patient's autonomy in matters of religion.

Many patients regard their religious faith as even more personal and private than their health. Religious practices can be disruptive as well as healing. Conflicts between Catholics & Protestants and among Christians, Jews & Muslims are evident at national levels in many countries.

Engaging patients in conversations about religious matters is not a simple process. Cultural and religious diversity is increasing rapidly in the United States. No doubt, many patients wish to obtain medical care from physicians who share their religious heritage but managed- care plans make this increasingly difficult by limiting the choice of a physician. Such patients can be appropriately referred to chaplains or clergy. The same applies to India and other countries.

Assessing the spirituality of patients and providing spiritual care require skill and at least an implied covenant between the provider and the recipient of such care. Evidence that patients want religion and spirituality to be incorporated into clinical medicine generally comes from studies in family practice settings, where physicians and patients are likely to know each other well. The degree to which patients express an interest in incorporating religion and spirituality into medical care depends on the clinical setting, the interpersonal and communication skills of the physician, the nature of the specific physician – patient relationship, and the characteristics of the patient. Patients often ask for things that are unrealistic or that may not be in their best interests. The decision by physicians to accede to their wishes is complex and requires weighing the conflicting ethical principles of beneficence and autonomy. The mere fact that some patients want physicians to address religious matters is not sufficient in itself to justify this practice.

Attempt to use religion instrumentally as one uses antibiotics or surgical procedures to treat diseases, may be deeply offensive to some people. If religion is considered only in its psychosocial dimension, it becomes indistinguishable from any other cultural practice.

Because the question of a link between religion and health care is so controversial, we must continue to address it, with discussions that cross disciplinary and specialty lines. Attempts should be made to obtain scientific evidence of the health benefits of religious activity. Religion is a spiritual way of being in the world.

Further there are certain methodological issues that pertain to research studies :

Confounders such as behavioral and genetic differences and stratification variables such as age, sex, education, ethnicity, socioeconomic status, and health status may have an important role in the association between religion and health. Failure to control for these factors can lead to a biased estimation of this association. For case control study, deficiencies are widely known. The strategy of matching ensures equivalence of groups only on the matched variables. As a consequence, the groups differed with respect to dietary habits, smoking, blood cholesterol concentrations and marital status, with the secular groups having greater risk. However, after control for all relevant covariates the relationship held valid only for women. Further, Pressman and colleagues reported that after surgical repair of broken hips, religiousness was associated with better ambulation status at discharge among elderly women only.

Many studies on religion and health fail to make an adjustment for the greater likelihood of finding a statistically significant result when conducting multiple statistical tests. There are similar problems in the published randomized clinical trial.

Durkheim's theory and the growing evidence suggesting a relationship between church or synagogue attendance and social support. Attendance at religious services has been associated with a sense of well-being, less depression, less anxiety and fewer suicides as well as lower blood pressure and longer survival rates. Comstock and Partridge reported that in 9-12 years follow-up study of 2754 community dwelling person aged 35-69 in the Tecumseh (Michigan) Community Health Study, frequent church attendance was significantly related to survival but only among women after age and health factor were controlled. Strabridge et al, however, observed that church attendance was associated with lower mortality, but only in women.

Inconsistencies also arise within studies not based on large epidemiological samples. For instance, while total cholesterol concentrations were lower across all age groups for a cohort of Seventh Day Adventists (SDA) than in age-matched healthy New York City men and women. Suggesting a lower risk of coronary hear disease among DSA, serum triglycerides of the SDA men in the coronary – prone age range (>32 years) were 19% higher than in the controls, which suggests the opposite. Though to some degree, lack of consistency is characteristic of an evolving field, inconsistency in the empirical findings makes it difficult to support recommendations for clinical interventions.

SPIRITUAL ASSESSMENT AND CARE

Developing an instrument to assess a client's spiritual needs is difficult because of the metaphysical nature of the elements of spirituality (Draper & McSherry, 2002). No single approach is likely to meet all the needs of all clients. Health care professionals increasingly recognize that clients want a holistic approach to their care and feel that their role is to "hear the patient into speech, to be a midwife of the spirit". It is important to be respectful of a broad range of world and religious views and to avoid a "one size-fits-all" perspective.

There are four steps to a systematic approach to spiritual care:-

1. **Assessing** the individual's spiritual status and identifying specific needs.
2. **Planning** mutually agreed-upon goals for action.
3. **Intervening and implementing** the planned actions.
4. **Evaluating** the individual's status after the intervention.

ASSESSMENT OF SPIRITUAL STATUS:

It provides a framework with which to identify the spiritual needs of a client. Difficulty may exist because spirituality in health care today is primarily being delivered from a Judeo-Christian perspective. Others, such as agnostics or atheists, may interpret spirituality from a more humanistic, existential perspective.

Multiple organizations mandate the assessment of spirituality. They are:-

1. Joint Commission on Accreditation of Health Care Organizations (JCAHO).
2. The World Health Organization (WHO).
3. The United Kingdom Central Council for Nurses, Midwives, and Health Visitors.
4. The American Nurses Association Code of Ethics.
5. The International Council of Nurses Code of Ethics for Nurses.
6. The American Association of Colleges of Nursing.
7. The Canadian Council on Health Services Accreditation.
8. American Psychological Association (APA).

According to JCAHO assessment should:-

1. Determine the patient's denomination, beliefs and spiritual practices.
2. Demonstrate respect for the person's values, religion and philosophy.
3. Include how and when pastoral care is requested and when to provide a list of spiritual resources in the community as well as spiritual leaders who are available on call.
4. Provide access to services that ensure religious freedom and availability of services to meet the person's spiritual needs.

Several fundamental actions should be completed before the spiritual assessment is undertaken. These actions include:-

1. Performing a spiritual self-assessment
2. Caring for the self in a spiritual way
3. Establishing a positive provider-client relationship
4. Appropriately timing the discussion about spirituality
5. Creating a "sacred space".

Performing a spiritual self-assessment allows health care professional to remain focused on the client and helps him or her remain non-judgmental when dealing with the client's specific spiritual concerns. It is done when they ask themselves following questions.

- Is faith important to me?
- Do I believe in God or a Higher Power?
- Do I participate in religious activities?
- Do I pray?
- Do I believe that spiritual care is an important component in providing health care?
- What strengths do I have to offer as a spiritual care provider?
- What areas do I need to strengthen in order to provide sensitive, compassionate spiritual care to my clients?

Additional Questions to be asked:

- What do I believe in?
- What gives my life meaning?
- What makes me smile?
- What is my favorite part of creation?
- If I could be anywhere, where would I be?
- What do I hope for?
- Who do I love and who loves me?
- When do I feel most connected to others?
- What is my understanding of spirituality?
- How do I express my spirituality?
- What relationship do I have with a Higher Being?
- Why is spiritual rituals care meaningful to me?
- What unique personal qualities can help me meet the spiritual needs of my clients?
- What client-care experiences have left me feeling uncomfortable or inadequate in the area of spiritual care?

Discomfort with any particular view or lifestyle does not make them unsuitable to provide spiritual care. An awareness of this discomfort and its causes can help health care professionals move past the discomfort and barriers and increase their self-awareness.

This can facilitate personal and spiritual growth and lead to better care of the professional and the client. Self awareness requires identification of feelings. Anger, jealously, grief and fear all have a purpose. For example, fear can help people be more cautious.

Bhay dikhaai le aavahu tat sakhaa sugriv (Shri Ram Charit Manas, Kiskindha Kand.......).

Similar is the case with Anger. *Bole Ram sakop tab.... bhaya binu hoi na preet (Shri Ram Charit Manas, Sunder Kand.......).*

Experts state that spirituality is not separate from daily life·

Caring for the self in a spiritual way can take many forms, including involvement in religious practices, community services activities, connecting with family and friends, spending time in natural suuroundings, meditating, participating in a favorite sport, or spending time alone.

Establishing a positive provider-client relationship starts with the understanding that spirituality is different from religiousness. Develop a sense of rapport and trust, in which a person feels free.

(Jo Aniti Kachhu Bhakhaun bhai, Tau Mohi Barjeu Bhaya Visarai) Shri Ram Charit Manas, Uttarkand, Doha-42, Chaupai-4.

Be an active listener – *Bed Puraan Vashisha Bakhanahi, Sunahi Ram Yadyapi Sab Jaanahi). (Ved Puraan sunahi man lai aap kahahi anuyahi samjhai) Shri Ram Charit Manas Ayodhya-204/3.*

Sharing personal experiences can be interpreted as imposing personal beliefs onto a client, or proselytizing, and may hinder communication. Explain the reasons for their inquiry and discuss with the client what they plan to do with the information obtained.

Appropriately timing the discussion about spirituality is crucial for the assessment. Take into consideration the client's overall status. If extremely ill, defer assessment. The appropriate time to address spiritual issues is judged by using Maslow's hierarchy of needs, which states that human beings are inclined to address their physical and safety needs before paying attention to mental and spiritual ones.

Often, a discussion of spiritual beliefs and practices flows naturally during a discussion of advanced directives, a new diagnosis of a severe, chronic, or terminal illness, end-of-life planning or during the grieving process. Ideally, a spiritual assessment should be an ongoing endeavor; the results may change over time.

Creating a "Sacred Space" is an important element. Sacred space is a place where one feels safe it can be created also. Any environment can be transformed into a sacred space by prayer, poetry, expression of love and concern, dance, rituals, the use of sound or music, candles, incense, the use of color, or through sacred or religious objects (e.g. art, crystals, pictures, or elements of nature). Every healing and caring act is a sacred act.

- Respect the person and his religious or spiritual behaviors.
- Focus on living rather than on illness and dying.
- Use positive nonverbal communication as a relaxing manner, leaning slightly toward the client, or an open posture where arms and legs are not crossed)

Questions may need to be modified or phrased in a way that considers cultural and educational backgrounds. Open-ended questions are the most effective (closed-ended questions if time is less).

Observation of nonverbal cues (especially facial expression) can provide information about any fear, doubt, depression or despair.

Numerous guides, instruments and scales are used to assess spirituality. The informal assessment can be accomplished at any time by carefully interpreting what the client is actually revealing using following questions (JCAHO 2001).

- Does the client use prayer in his/her life?
- How does the client express his or her spirituality?
- What type of spiritual / religious support does the client require?
- How does the client describe his or her philosophy of life?
- What are the client's spiritual goals?
- Is a belief in God important to the client?
- What are the names of the client's clergy, ministers, chaplains, pastors, rabbis?
- How has the illness affected the client and his or her family?
- How does faith help the client keep going the health care experience?

For formal assessment, tools need to be easy to use, flexible, optimally quick, nonintrusive, use encouraging words, should not interrogate, alienate or discriminate between various religious groups, to be conducted in a nonthreatening nonjudgmental manner.

There are several formal assessment tools including. Howden's spirituality assessment scale which is "designed to measure spirituality understood as the integrating or unifying dimension of our being". It addressed four specific areas- purpose and meaning life, innerness or inner resources, unifying interconnectedness and transcendence; the FICA model, (faith and belief, importance and influence of faith and beliefs, community, and address in care) and *JAREL spiritual well-being scale*, being *most comprehensive is meant to inquire about following:*

1. Prayer is an important part of life.
2. I believe I have spiritual well-being.
3. As I grow older, I find myself more tolerant of others beliefs.
4. I find meaning and purpose in my life.
5. I feel there is a close relationship between my spiritual beliefs and what I do.
6. I believe in an afterlife.
7. When I am sick, I have less spiritual well-being.
8. I believe in a supreme being.
9. I am able to receive and give love to others.
10. I am satisfied with my life.
11. I set goals for myself.
12. God has little meaning in my life.
13. I am satisfied with the way I am using my abilities.
14. Prayer does not help me in making decisions.
15. I am able to appreciate differences in others.
16. I am pretty well put together.
17. I prefer that others make decision for me.
18. I find it hard to forgive others.
19. I accept my life situations.
20. Belief in a supreme being has no part in my life.
21. I cannot accept change in my life.

A still better spiritual assessment tool which includes open-ended, reflective questions that can assist health care providers in developing a deeper spiritual awareness for themselves and others can be found in *Spirituality: Living Our Connectedness*.

The qualitative assessment tools, which give maximum "room for clients to negotiate a shared understanding of the individual experiences" since it also includes taking a spiritual history (similar to taking a family history).

The patient's narration is then interpreted as follows:-

1. Affect: How does their spirituality affects life today?
2. Behavior: In what ways do they practice their spirituality?
3. Cognition: What are their current beliefs and how do they affect their life?
4. Communication: What is their experience with the Ultimate?
5. Conscience: How does their spirituality determine right and wrong, impact their key values, and help them deal with guilt and sin?
6. Intuition: Have hunches, premonitions, or spiritual insights affected their life?

The aim of assessment is to rule out spiritual distress specific characteristics which include the following:-

- Questions about the moral / ethical implications of a therapeutic regimen.
- Feelings of worthlessness, bitterness, denial, guilt and fear.
- Nightmares and sleep disturbances.
- Anorexia.
- Somatic complaints.
- Verbalization of inner conflicts about beliefs.
- Inability to participate in usual religious practices.
- Seeking of spiritual assistance.
- Questioning the meaning of suffering.
- Questioning the meaning of one's existence.
- Anger toward God.
- Alterations in mood / behavior (anger, crying, withdrawal, anxiety, apathy, etc).
- Gallows humor.

Risk factors for spiritual distress include the following:-

- Medical illness or impending death.
- Loss of a loved one.
- Low self-esteem.
- Mental illness.
- Natural disaster.
- Physical illness.
- Situational losses.
- Substance abuse.
- Poor relationship with others.

- Physical or psychological stress.
- Inability to forgive (either the self or others).
- Lack of self-love.
- Extreme anxiety.

The care for a person in spiritual distress can be achieved by implementing specific interventions such as the following:

- Determining the spiritual or religious orientation and influence of the client's and family's belief systems.
- Noting expressions of the inability to find meaning in life.
- Listening to expressions of anger or alienation from God.
- Providing a sacred space for the individual to express his concerns.
- Expressing acceptance of the client's beliefs.
- Asking how you might be most helpful to the client.
- Developing a therapeutic relationship with the client and the family.
- Helping the client and the family find spiritual / religious resources and support.

Additional diagnosis in the form of spiritual pain (the expression of discomfort or suffering related to one's experience with God), spiritual alienation (the feeling that God seems very far away or remote from one's everyday life), spiritual anxiety (a fear that God is displeased with the individuals behavior), spiritual guilt (a fear that the individual has failed to do the things that should be done in a spiritual life, spiritual anger (frustration, anguish or outrage directed at God for allowing trials, sickness or perceived unfairness), spiritual loss (a feeling of emptiness regarding spiritual matters) and spiritual despair (a feeling that God no longer cares) should also be made.

Once the assessment has been completed, the information gained can be used to formulate an effective plan of spiritual care based on needs identified during assessment phase. Spiritual care giving can include four areas:-

1. Affirmation: The acknowledgement of factors in a client life that could be considered positive.
2. Therapeutic communication: "Listening" to the meaning of the client's conversation through (clever) observation of body language and facial expression and through maintaining an active "presence" with the client.

3. Reminiscence: A life review that allows the client to discuss people, places, or situations that is / was meaningful in her life.
4. Referral: The appropriate recommendation to a spiritual health care provider, such as clergy.

Several option may be considered-allowing the client time to pray or read in private, arranging care so that the client can attend a religious service, or contacting the clients religious or spiritual leaders for support, helping the client work through spiritual issues with a chaplain or spiritual leader or providing information about adviser or medicine man to conduct specific spiritual rituals for the client. Modify the treatment plan as needed once the spiritual needs of the client are understood.

Implementing spiritual care requires committing energy and time to the goals, which may mean conversations at night when many clients may feel more willing to discuss these types of issues than during the daytime. Interventions can include the following actions:-

- Caring touch – *Kar parsaa sugriv sariraa, tan bhaa kulis gari sab pira (Shri Ram Charit Manas, Kiskindha Kand, doha no.7, Chaupai. No.3).*
- Analysing dreams – *Sapne Vaanar Lankaajaani, Jatudhan sena sab maari (Sunder Kand, doha no. 10, Chaupai No. 2).*
- Reading spiritually uplifting materials, including sacred writings.
- Utilizing art as a means of expressing spiritual thoughts and beliefs.
- Facilitating the use of spiritual rituals.
- Utilizing humor – *Bilag-Bilag hoi chalahun baraataa, Hansi karaiu par pur jaataa (Shri Ram Charit Manas, Ballkand).*
- Utilizing imagery, meditation, or prayer.
- Encouraging journal writing or scrapbook making.
- Encouraging experiences in nature – *Param ramya uttam yah dharani, Mahimaa amit jai nahi barani (Shri Ram Charit Manas, Lanka Kand).*
- Incorporating storytelling, reminiscing, or life review into care plans.
- Using institution.

- Behavioral interventions.

Health care professionals should recognize and understand their own limitations and utilize other available professional resources whenever and wherever appropriate.

Evaluating spiritual care is a final difficult step since spiritual dimension is a subjective one. It can be quite difficult to measure cause and effect as they relate to a spiritual intervention. Consultation with the client and participation in the interventions are two factors that help determine their effectiveness. Perhaps the most obvious way to measure the effectiveness of spiritual intervention is to ask the client directly, and carefully observe her physical, verbal, or nonverbal cues. For example, the health care provider can observe whether a client attends a particular service or document that the client's spiritual / religious leader came to visit.

One difficulty with evaluating whether or not spiritual goals were achieved is the time frame involved in achieving them. It may take an individual many months to resolve a health problem or personal crisis. It is unrealistic to expect a client to reflect, adjust and regain her spiritual balance in a matter of hours, days or even weeks. Thus, the specific spiritual needs of a client should be carefully considered and time frames for implementation and evaluation of spiritual goals realistically decided. Finally every thing must be documented which will help in sharing knowledge, auditing, quality assurance and conducting research.

Spirituality becomes almost tangible when individuals face crises, emotional stress, physical illness, or death and is often the very force that provides health care with the strength to face the daily challenges of their profession.

Spiritual health care providers by client's preference in descending order are family and friends, personal clergy, physicians, nurses, chaplains, psychiatrists or psychologists, and social workers. Nurses, physicians, and social workers are *spiritual care generalists*, while chaplains, clergy, parish nurses, spiritual mentors, family and friends and folk healers are considered *spiritual care specialists.*

Female nurse, Florence Nightingale was the first to believe that spirituality was an essential part of human nature and the most potent resource for healing and also that science was the basis for a relationship with God. She believed that the focus of nursing was to create an environment in which natural healing might take place. This environment included cleanliness, fresh air, and sunlight, and warmth, quiet and proper nutrition. Nursing is a manifestation of God's love expressed through caring, compassion and charity toward the sick and the poor. Nursing saw the patient as a "whole" and treated her holistically. Nightingale recognized a force that healed and was greater than herself. Nursing, comprised mostly of women, has been increasingly felt as subordinate to physicians, who were mostly male. It needs to be curbed.

The physician-client relationship, like that of other health care providers with their clients, is essentially a spiritual relationship. Many clients wish their physicians would talk to them about spiritual matters, pray them or draw on spiritual coping resources during times of crisis. During one survey at a meeting of the American Academy of Family Physicians, 99% of physicians stated they believed religious beliefs can heal and 75% believed that the prayers of others can aid in healing. Yet, most of these physicians also reported that they rarely discussed spiritual issues with their clients. As more and more physicians receive training in spiritual area and study the results of research on the importance of spirituality in health, they will assume a more active role in the spiritual care process.

Social workers may assist in the spiritual care process in many ways, including helping families organize their care support system and guiding the client and family in meeting their emotional, spiritual, and psychological and bereavement needs.

Folk healing systems are "a formal, coherent and consistent set of beliefs and practices ascribed to a particular culture". Here, knowledge is passed from one generation to another. The folk or lay healers focus on a holistic framework that promotes harmony rather than diagnosis and curing. They use techniques unique to their culture have specific attributes and a defined status within their culture. They may use special rituals, herbs or other natural materials to promote health and they usually receive their education as the result of an apprenticeship, personal study, or experience. Their cultural practices are justified because they deal routinely with social, psychological, physical, and spiritual issues that are often ignored by conventional physicians (Trotter 2001). Some believe that certain folk healing beliefs and practices, such as healing, holism, and therapeutic touch, are the "very essence of contemporary nursing". The use of local remedies is only one aspect of folk healing. Another equally important aspect is the meaning assigned to sickness and the beliefs and act associated with the special ministrations. The cultures that use folk healers often consider sickness the result of a sin; God's punishment; casual agents such as lighting, water or wind (Navajo Indians). Shamans act as a guide to the soil (Rhi 2001;P-569). Folk healers may utilize many types of activities to support their client on the journey to total well-being. These include the following :-

- Affirmations
- Visualizations
- A positive attitude
- Relaxation and stress reduction techniques.
- Healing energy.
- Supporting positive relationships in the client,s life.
- Encouraging time in nature.
- Meditation.
- Visual arts to represent the holy people in their human form.
- Music.
- Healing ceremonies.
- Connecting with God or a higher power.
- Faith, prayer and hope.

Folk healers – especially curanderos – often conceal their identity to the members of the outside culture. Barriers to providing spiritual care are: - lack of education, lack of time, lack of privacy, fear of invading a clients privacy, worry about the inappropriateness, lack of proper method, fear of being misjudged, inability to communicate due to an illness or loss of sense, own prejudices about care and behaviors.

VALIDATION OF WOMEN SPIRITUAL HELP-SEEKING BEHAVIOUR MEASURE (WSHBM):

Recent research findings revealed that more women than men seek help from spiritual houses, yet little is known regarding the type of problems that women seek spiritual help for. African's believe in spirits and the supernatural has reflected in their help-seeking behavior, therefore their preference for spiritual houses and not formal help centers. Despite the volume of available researches in the area of women help-seeking, there is no known indigenous help-seeking behavior measure that could be used particularly to assess women's spiritual help-seeking behavior. It is believed that Women Spiritual Help-Seeking Behaviour Measure can be useful in helping psychologist, counselors and help-givers in carrying out easy and valid assessment of the help-seekers. Using a systematic random sampling procedure 500 women help-seekers aged 17-69 years old were sampled. This sample was drawn from 8 help-giving centers that were identified snowballing sampling technique. The scale has a Cronbach's Alpha reliability coefficient of 0.97 and Guttmann split half reliability of .90. The factor structure of the scale was extracted by performing principal component analysis with varimax rotation which showed that Women Spiritual Help-Seeking Behavior Measure has a five factor structure (Family, Health, Carrier, Finance and Persecutory). Study findings showed that Women Spiritual Help-Seeking Behavior Measure has a good structural characteristic and is a reliable and valid instrument that can be used for measuring women spiritual help-seeking behavior.

MORAL AND ETHICAL ISSUSES IN SPIRITUAL CARE

Mortality, ethics and spirituality are inextricably related and intertwined with culture, religion, values, emotions, and the social aspects of an individual. Health care professionals find their origin, purpose, and meaning within the context of culturally accepted moral norms, individual values, and perceived social nee.

- Mortality deals with what is "good" or "bad", "right" or "wrong". It refers to the "rules a society has created for promoting ethical conduct or right and virtuous behavior".
- Ethics is concerned with what one "ought" or "should" do in any given situation, and it is the process by which motality is practised.
- Values contain potent emotional and spiritual significance and are powerful determinants of behavior. Ethical questions such as "what is the right thing for me to do?" raise spiritual questions such as "what is of value to me?"

If health care professionals truly believe in the holistic concept of client care, they have an ethical obligation to provide spiritual care. The words health, holy and whole is derived from the old Saxon word "Hal" and the Greek "holos", which mean "Whole." Thus, by their nature, then, health and healing are associated with that which is holy and whole.

The major ethical principles of beneficence, nonmaleficence, autonomy, confidentiality and advocacy apply to the spiritual care of clients. They may be helpful in assisting health care professionals when they encounter such questions as the following:

- What should I do if the client or family invites me to pray with them?
- How can I give spiritual care without unduly influencing the client or the family?
- Can I give spiritual care if a client or family is of a different faith or religion?
- Should I initiate prayer for a client or family?
- Is it unethical to pray for a client without his or her consent?

Beneficence (i.e. the duty to do the right thing) obligates the health care provider to act in a positive way to benefit the client.

Nonmaleficence (i.e. the duty to do no harm to a client) It can be interpreted to mean that a health care professional must provide spiritual care as part of the overall care, since withholding spiritual care can negatively impact the client. Clients regard their spiritual health and physical health as equally important.

Autonomy means "self governing" or self-determination" and in relation to spiritual care can be interpreted to mean assisting clients with their spiritual needs without imposing one's own beliefs on that client.

Confidentiality is the ethical principle that requires individuals who are entrusted with private or secret information to keep that information private or secret.

Finally, advocacy involves helping *clients exercise their autonomy*. It requires the health care professional to "*honor the dignity and freedom of the patient in a convenient relationship as modeled between God and believers*". The spiritual care provider who is a client advocate is able to set aside his or her personal agendas and help clients search for their own meaning during times of suffering, frustration and vulnerability.

Jadapi sakhaa tab itchhaa naahi, Mor Daras Amogh Jagmaahi.

As kahi ram lilak tehi saaraa, suman vrasti navh bhai apaaraa (Shri Ram Charit Manas, Sunderkand).

Many experts believe that since spirituality can not be measured, it might not be ethical to assist clients with their spiritual needs when health care providers cannot measure the impact of that intervention and that it will be deemed to be coercive since the relationship between clients and provider is unequal. Spirituality is an important part of wellness and an indispensable care. Therefore, professional and ethical obligations oblige health care providers to develop their skills in the delivery of spiritual care.

Spirituality, which pertains to ultimate meaning and purpose in life, has clinical relevance. Patients are especially concerned with spirituality in the context of suffering, debilitation and dyeing. For some patients, these concerns may be taken up entirely within the context of human relations, values and purpose; for others, their resolution involves faith in a higher being in the universe, one that is a source of reassurance and hope. Why address spirituality as a matter of serious medical and ethical concern? It can attract more patients to proven interventions. Anxiety and hope can be factors in illness outcomes, the keys for which are frequently found within the matrix of patient's spirituality. Deciding how best to respond to a patient's spiritual commitments; however, can raise professional ethical issues for physicians. Should physicians discuss spiritual issues? Is it ever appropriate to try to encourage or discourage religious beliefs for the "benefit" of the patient? What should be the professional boundaries between physicians and chaplains, who can be clergy or nonclergy lay persons with clinical pastoral education? Should an appreciation of patient spirituality also be expressed within the physician-patients relationship? If so, under what circumstances and to what extent should it be done? Although it is true that, historically, some persons have been trained as both a religious clergy person and as a physician (for example, Rabbi-physicians such as Moses Maimonides and the colonial American clergy-physicians), it is a general mandate of modern developed societies to keep the professional roles separate. In most of the societies, religious traditions (and, therefore, many patients) still regard the physicians as both the skilled agent of scientifically informed clinical interventions and as an instrument of a higher healing power. When the healer was less able to intervene in disease, the patient's knowledge of the physician's divine backdrop could enhance the potential placebo effect by increasing patient belief and confidence, thereby enabling some patients to heal themselves. Professional's boundaries may appear somewhat artificial to the patient who believes that God is working through the physician. This does not mean that these boundaries are unimportant. The pressure to blur the boundaries between the professions often comes from patients.

Adding a sacred or religious mystique to the power of the physician is suspect. Around 48% of patients want prayer with their physicians and 64% of Americans think that physicians should join their patients in prayer if the patients ask. Physicians initiated prayers 53% of the time. A physician who initiates a prayer without first being asked presents an ethical concern in that patients might easily feel coerced. It argues, that the prayer should be led by an "identified religious leader distinct from the treating medical team whenever possible. Physician led Prayer is acceptable only when pastoral care is not readily available, when the patient is intent on prayer with the physicians, and when the physician can pray without having to feign faith and without manipulating the patient.

Immanuel Jakobovits, Chief Rabbi of the British Commonwealth of Nations, wrote that "Diseases forges an especially close link between God and Man; the Divine Presence Itself, as it were 'rests on the head of sickbed". Those standing around the sickbed – the patient's family, physicians, and chaplain – will all relate to that presence in different ways. As the health care market presses providers in a more holistic direction that include *attentiveness to patient spirituality*, we expect that the ethical issues that we are beginning to address here will become even more significant in the standard clinical setting.

RELIGION AND PUBLIC HEALTH INTERVENTION

Women of color can be helped to embrace their spirituality to facilitate health promotion, healing and coping through spirituality insight and reflection as well as religious practice. Health and healing aspects within women' faith traditions can promote positive behaviors. For example, various faith traditions enjoin their adherents to make dietary and other lifestyle choices that are beneficial, such as practicing sexual responsibility and abstaining from tobacco and alcohol.

The spiritual, physical, mental and social aspects of the Hispanic health concept were explicitly acknowledged by the planners, who included a religious service, a communal lunch, several health- related presentations, and screening for diabetes, hypertension, and vision problems.

For example, a faith based program to train cancer survivors to promote increased mammography and breast self-examination among rural African American women (the Witness Project) has led to significant increases in breast self-examination and mammogrpahy. The HIV prevention faith initiative of the Centers for Disease Control and Prevention is a government and faith-based partnership between the surgeon general, the Congressional Black Caucus, and gospel artists, who work together to dispel myths and encourage audience take HIV tests. Religious leaders are trusted by and religious institutions reach people from all walks of life, especially hard-to- reach populations.

The experience of a Black woman whose son was diagnosed with HIV illustrates the multilayered integration of spirituality and health. First, she relied on her spirituality and the support of her faith community for personal sustenance. Next, she sensitized fellow congregants to HIV/AIDS and provided health education. Finally she mobilized a group within the church to provide compassionate care to AIDS victims from diagnosis to their deaths.

Spirituality and religiosity are of significant benefit to women who are experiencing challenges to their health and well being. The implications for prevention, health behaviors, and coping with health problems are evident. The intersection of spirituality or religiosity and health for ethnic women of color can make a difference in their health experience, helping to eliminate health disparities and promoting positive health outcomes.

References

1. Caroline Young & Cyndie Koopsen. Spirituality, Health & Healing. Jones & Bartlett Publisher. United States, 2005.
2. Reed PG. Spirituality and mental health in older adults: extant knowledge for nursing. Fam Community Health. 1991;14(2):14-25.
3. Christ C. Spirituality for Women: In: Christ C, ed. Laughter of Aphrodite: Reflections on a Journey to the Goddess. New York: Harper Collins;1987.

4. Gross RM. Feminism & Religion: An Introduction Boston: Beacon Press: 1996.
5. Johnson RA, Wallwork E, Green C, Santmire HP, Vanderpool HY. Paul Tillich: the relative and the ultimate in the encounter of religious. In: Johnson RA, Wallwork E, Green C, Santmire HP, Vanderpool HY, eds. Critical Issues in Modern Religious. Englewood Cliffs, NJ:Prentice Hall; 1973.
6. www.alleghenyreproducive.com/promiting _spiritual_health.html accessed on 10.03.08
7. Ito T, Cacioppo J. Representation of the contours of positive human health. Psychol Inquiry, 1998;9(1):43-48.
8. Ryff C, Singer B. The contours of positive human health. Psychol Inquiry, 1998;9:1-28.
9. Ruzek S, Olesen V, Clarke A eds. Women's Health: Complexities and Differences. Columbus, OH: Ohio State University Press:1993.
10. Reis HR, Frank P. The role of intimacy and social support in health outcomes: two processes or one? Personal Relationships. 1994;1:185-197.
11. Writing Group of the 1996 AAN Expert Panel on Women's Health. Women's health and women's health care: recommendations of the 1996 AAN Expert Panel on Women's Health. Nurs Outlook. 1997;45:7-15.
12. Diane Ruth Lauver, Commonalities in Women's Spirituality & Women's Health. Advances in Nursing Science 2000;22(3):276-88.
13. Sheilds LE. Women's experiences of the meaning of empowerment. Qual Health Res. 1995;5(1):15-35.
13. Pollner M. Divine relations, social relations, and well-being. J Health Soc Behav 1989;30:92-104.
14. Weisman C. Women's Health Care: Activist Traditions and Institutional Change. Baltimore: Johns Hopkins University Press; 1998.
15. Schaps MJ, Linn ES, Wilbanks GD, Silbanks ER. Women-centered care: Implementing a philosophy. Wom Health Issues. 1993;3(2):52-54.
16. Tillich P. The meaning of health. In: LeFever P ed. The meaning of Health: Essays in Existentialism, Psychoanalysis and Religion. Chicago: Exploration Press; 1984.
17. Reed P. Self-transcendence and mental health in oldest old adults. Nurs Res. 1991;40(1):5-11.

18. Kass JD, Friedman R, Leserman J, Zuttermeister PC, Benson H. Health outcomes and a new index of spiritual experience. J Sci Study Religion. 1991;30:203-212.
19. Ryan RM, Rigby S, King K. Two types of religious internalization and their relations to religious orientations and mental health. J Pers Soc Psychol. 1991;65:586-596.
20. Plaskow J, Christ CP, eds. Weaving the Visions: New patterns in Feminist Spirituality. San Francisco: Harper & Row; 1989.
21. Procter-Smith M, Walton JR, eds. Women at Worship: Interpretations of North American Diversity. Louisville KY: Westminister / John Knox Press; 1993.
22. Kabat-Zinn J. Wherever You Go, There You Are: Mindfulness Mediation I Everyday Life. New York: Hyperion Press; 1994.
23. Kornfield J. A Path with Heart: A Guide through the perils and promises of spiritual life. New York: Bantam Books; 1993.
24. Hellman CJ, Budd M, Borysenko J, McLelland DC, Benson H. A study of the effectiveness of two group behavioural medicine interventions for patients with psycho-somatic complaints. Behav Med 1990;16:165-173.
25. Cimprich B. Development of an intervention to restore attention in cancer patients. Cancer Nurs 1993;16(2):83-92.
26. Northrup C. Women's Bodies, Women's Wisdom. New York: Bantam Books; 1994.
27. Neu DL. Women's empowerment through feminist rituals. In: Ochshorn J, Cole E eds. Women's Spirituality, Women's Lives. New York: Haworth Press; 1995.
28. Achterberg J, Dossey B, Kolkmeier L. Rituals of Healing: Using Imagery for Health and Wellness. New York. Bantam Books; 1994.
29. www.experiencefestival.com/a/womens_spirituality/id/3626 accessed on 20.02.08.
30. www.aafp.org/afp/20010101/81.html accessed on 20.02.08.
31. Musgrave et al. Am J Pub Health, 2002;92(4):557-560.
32. Higgins PG, Learn CD. Health practices of adult Hispanic women. J Adv Nurs 1999;29:1105-1112.
33. Zorn CR, Johnson MT. Religious well-being in nonistitutionalized elederly women. Health Care Women Int. 1997;18:209-219.
34. Zhan L, Cloutterbuck J, Keshian I, Lombardi L. Promoting health: Perspectives from ethnic elderly women. J Community Health Nurs. 1998;15:31-44.

35. Somali AM, Heckman TG, Hadd K et al. Developments stages and spiritual coping responses women living with HIV disease. J Pastoral Care. 1998;52:227-240.
36. Siegel K, Schrimshaw EW. Presenting benefits in adversity: stress related growth in women living with HIV/AIDS. Soc Sci Med 2000;51:1543-1554.
37. Catherine I.O'Connor. Characteristics of spirituality, assessment and prayer. Holistic Nursing.2001;36 (1):33-46.
39. Dennis Patrick O'Hara. Is there a role for prayer and spirituality in health care? Medical clinics of North America. 2002:86,1.
40. Levin JS. Religion and health: is there an association, is it valid and is casual? Soc Sci Med. 1994 ; 38 : 1475-82.
41. Koening HG, Idler E, Kasl S, Hays JC, George LK, Musick M et al. Religion., Spirituality and Medicine: a rebuttal to skeptics. Int J psychiatry Med. 1999:29:123-31
42. Levin JS, Larson DB, Puchalski CM. Religion and spirituality in Medicine, research and education. JAMA.1997;278:792-3
43. Durkheim E. The elementary forms of religious experience. London: Allen & Unwin 1915.
44. Comstock GW, Partidge KB. Church attendance in health. J Chron Dise 1972;24:665- 672.
45. Strawbridge WJ, Cohen RD, Shema SJ, Kaplan GA. Frequent attendance at religious services and mortality over 28 years. Am J Pub Heal 1997;87:957-961.
46. Draper P & McSherry W. A critical view of spirituality and spiritual assessment. *Journal of Dossey BM. Florence Nightingale*: Mystic, visionary, healer. Springhouse, PA: Springhouse 2000. Advanced Nursing 002;39(1):1-2.
47. Benedict LM. Spiritual assessment: EDA 318-0479. Carrollton, TX: PRIMEDIA Healthcare: Long-term care network.2002.
48. Joint Commission on Accreditation of Healthcare Organizations. Spiritual assessment retrieved June 16, 2002.
49. Govier I. Spiritual care in nursing: A systematic approach. Nursing Standards 2000;14(17):32- 36.
50. Burkhard MA & Nagai-Jacobson MG. Spirituality: Living our connectedness. 2002, New York: Delmar Thomson Learning.
51. Shri Ramcharit Manas by Sant Tulsi Das, Gita Press Gorakhpur.
52. Taylor EJ. Spiritual care: Upper Saddle River, NJ: Prentice Hall 2002.

53. Wright SG & Sayre-Adams J. Sacred space: Right relationship and spirituality in healthcare. London: Harcourt Publishers Limited 2000.
54. Brush BL & Daly PR. Assessing spirituality in primary care practice: Is there time?Clinical Excellence for Nurse Practitioners 2000;4(2):67-71.
55. O' Neill PA. Caring for the older adult: A health promotion perspective. Philadelpha: WB Saunders 2002.
56. Dossey BM, Keegan L & Guzzetta CE. Holistic Nursing: A handbook for practice 2000;3rd Ed. Gaithersburg MD: Aspen.
57. Boudreaux ED, O'Hea E & Chasuk R. Spiritual role in healing: An alternative way of thinking. Primary Care: Clinics in Office Practice 2002;29(2):439-454.
58. Larson DB & Koenig HG. Is God good for your health? The role of spirituality in medical care. Cleveland Clinic Journal of Medicine 2000;67(2):80-84.
59. Larimore WL. Providing basic spiritual care for patients: Should it be the exclusive domain of pastroal professionals? American Family Physician 2001;67(2):80-84.
60. O'Hara DP. Is there a role for prayer and spirituality in health care? Medical Clinics of North America 2002;86(1),vi:33-46.
61. Rhi BY. Culture, spirituality, and mental health: The forgotten aspect of religion and health. Psychiatric Clinics of North America 2001;24(3), ix-x: 569-579.
62. Zapata J & Shippee-Rice R. The use of folk healing and healers by six Latinos living in New England: A preliminary study. Journal of Transcultural Nursing. 1999;19(2):136-142.
63. Oladipo SE. Development and Validation of women spiritual heal-seeking behaviour measure (WSHBM). J Soc Sci 2008;16(3):183-186.
64. Burkhardt MA & Nathaniel AK. Ethics and issues: New York: Delmar Thomson Learning 1998.
65. Treloar, LL (2001). Is spiritual care ethical? Journal of Christian Nursing, 18(2), 16-20.
66. Mueller, P.S., Plevak, D.J. & Rummans, T.A. (2001). Religious involvement, spirituality and medicine: Implications for clinical practice. Mayo Clinic Proceedings 76(12), 1225-1235.
67. Erwin DO, Spatz TS et al. Increasing mammography practice by African American women. Cancer Practice 1999;7:78-85.

68. Quander L. Faith-based program fight HIV/AIDS in minority communities. HIV Impact. Winter 2000;1-2.

38

Urinary Incontinence – Behavior Therapy for Urine Leakage

Santosh Kumari, Amarjeet Singh, Vanita Jain and A. K. Mandal

Urinary incontinence (U.I.) is one of the most common health problem affecting millions of women worldwide. The involuntary loss of urine can vary from the occasional nuisance of losing a few drops of urine to a more serious problem of losing larger amount of urine several times a day. Urinary incontinence is often severe enough to have significant social and/or hygienic consequences for women. It is a major clinical problem in most obstetric/gynecology departments. It affects all age groups and is particularly common among elderly. Approximately 15-30% of older women suffer from urinary incontinence. In two studies conducted in North India urinary incontinence was reported in 40% and 54% of uterine prolapse cases, with a population prevalence of 3.1% and 5.2% for stress incontinence among women 18 years and above. In a study from Chandigarh prevalence of 11.6% was detected. Prevalence studies show that urinary incontinence is endemic among women of every age group. Overall, irrespective of definition, the reported prevalence was at least 30% i.e. almost 1/3rd of women suffer from urinary incontinence.

Incontinent individuals are often reluctant to seek help because they view it as a normal part of the aging process. Many do not report the problem until they have had the symptoms for a long time. Unfortunately, those who do seek help frequently do not receive the attention they deserve. Incontinence remains largely a neglected problem despite the fact that it is treatable and often curable. Urinary incontinence is a chronic health problem which severely reduces the quality of life of women. It is an embarrassing symptom which is grossly under-reported by women.

Types of incontinence

Stress incontinence: This is an involuntary loss of urine on exertion, e.g. coughing, sneezing, and running, laughing and jumping. Leakage occurs when there is increase in intra-abdominal pressure caused by physical activities. It is most common in younger women and the second most common in elderly women and is also known as outlet incompetence. It is usually due to pelvic muscle or ligament laxity. Small volume of urine is usually lost.

Urge incontinence: This term is used to define the symptoms that result from involuntary contractions of the bladder muscle which may occur spontaneously. A patient with urge incontinence usually reports the loss of large volume of urine with each episode of incontinence. If a person does not reach toilet in time, urine leak occurs.

Mixed incontinence: In this type of incontinence the symptoms of both stress incontinence and urge incontinence are present.

Risk factors for urinary incontinence:

(a) Predisposing Factors:

Gender:

Women are at least thrice as likely to suffer from incontinence as compared to males. A female to male ratio of approximately 4:1 exists at ages below 60 years and a ratio of 2:1 occurs at age 60 years and older.

Age:

Prevalence of urinary incontinence increases with age. Prevalence of incontinence increases with age. After the age of 40 yrs incontinence is 2-4 times more common. In a study, the UI prevalence of 3.4% in age group 20-24 yrs. increased to 23.7% in people aged 65 years and above. Age more than 75 years has 70% increased risk for urinary incontinence.

Race:

A very low prevalence of UI was reported (4.5%) from Singapore, suggesting the ethnic advantage of studied group. The racial difference in the investigation revealed an incontinence rate of 1.1% for Malay Singaporeans, 1.6% for Indian and 5.2% for Chinese Singaporians. Indian females are more prone to develop stress urinary incontinence as compared to Black women. It was reported that Pakistani females using commode type of toilet had a higher incontinence (28.5%) than those voiding in squatting position (12.3%).

(b) Inciting Factors:

Radical pelvic surgery and radiation are identifiable as inciting factors for pelvic floor dysfunction, but are applicable to only a small subset of women. Clearly, vaginal delivery is the major inciting factor for the development of pelvic floor dysfunction in the majority of women.

Parity:

Most studies show significantly increased risks for urinary incontinence related to parity. Parity 3 or above has twice the risk.

Vaginal Childbirth:

Urinary incontinence and stress urinary incontinence is strongly associated with vaginal childbirth.

Forceps delivery or instrumental delivery has been reported as risk factor for urinary incontinence, when compared with those women who had normal delivery.

Heavy weight of children delivered by vaginal delivery and a wider circumference of fetal head also has been reported to predispose to prolapsed uterus.

Several studies have shown that prevalence of stress urinary incontinence increased during pregnancy and declined after delivery.

In a study from UK stress urinary incontinence during pregnancy was 43.7% and postnatal prevalence was 14.8%. In another study from Denmark stress urinary incontinence during pregnancy was 32% and it was 3% one year after delivery. Among women who reported stress incontinence (SUI) during pregnancy, less than 5% remained incontinent one year after delivery. In contrast, among women who reported onset of SUI after delivery 24% remained symptomatic after one year. This indicates that the increased pressure from the growing uterus on the bladder may cause temporary leakage during pregnancy. The women who have onset of symptoms after delivery are at increased risk for urinary incontinence in later life.

(c) Promoting Factors:

Promoting factors are the ones which aggravate the already existing urinary incontinence.

Constipation:

There is a growing body of evidence linking chronic constipation with urinary incontinence, fecal incontinence and pelvic organ prolapsed (2-13 times higher risk).

Occupational and Recreational Stresses:

Most reports have reported a higher prevalence of Incontinence in athletes.

Obesity:

Obesity is a commonly cited risk factor related to the development and recurrence of urinary incontinence in women.(2-3 times higher risk)

Surgery: Hysterectomy has twice the risk of UI.

Chronic Lung Disease and Smoking:

The relationship between cigarette smoking and chronic respiratory problem is irrefutable. Smokers are likely to develop persistent cough and stress urinary incontinence. Those who suffer from chronic lung disease are more likely to develop stress urinary incontinence. More violent coughing promotes the earlier development of the anatomic and pressure transmission defect leading to stress urinary incontinence. Due to cough, there is increase in intra-abdominal pressure which is transmitted to bladder and urethra which is unable to sustain adequate pressure under exertional circumstances.

Infection:-

Evidence suggests that acute urinary tract infection is associated with acute urinary incontinence of both stress and urge variety in about 1/4th of the infected women. Successful treatment of infection has been shown to relieve urge and stress incontinence. A history of previous urinary tract infection has been significantly associated with urge urinary incontinence.

Menopause:

Menopause and estrogen depletion leads to atrophy of mucosal tissue that lines both urethra and vagina. It results in weak urethra and reduces urethral pressure. In a study it was revealed that women with stress urinary incontinence have an altered tissue metabolism causing decreased collagen production, which may result in insufficient support of urogenital tract. Urinary incontinence has been reported to be more prevalent among menopausal women. Postmenopausal hormonal replacement appears to increase the risk of developing urinary incontinence.

(C) Decompensating Factors:

A variety of factors extrinsic to the pelvic floor and independent of changes in pelvic floor structure or function cause the compensated, although less than perfect, patient to decompensate and become symptomatic.

Some medicines like non-steroidal anti-inflammatory drugs, calcium containing antacids, or iron can cause constipation and predispose the patients to urinary incontinence. Some drugs can cause severe nonproductive cough. Diuretics can cause more production of urine and it becomes difficult for older patients to reach toilet in time. Decreased mobility may prevent an otherwise compensated individual for going to toilet in time leading to urinary incontinence. Co—morbid conditions such as diabetes, vascular insufficiency or congestive heart failure may overwhelm fragile continence reserve with a sudden increase in urine output. Diabetes as a risk factor has been reported by some studies. Hypertension as risk factor for urinary incontinence has also been reported. Arthritis has been reported to be associated with urinary incontinence. Arthritis patients are 70% more prone to urinary incontinence.

An association between high caffeine intake and detrusor instability has been found. Family history of urinary incontinence is also reported by some studies as a risk factor. The relatives of incontinent women displayed a higher prevalence of SUI (71.4%) among mothers and (24.6%) among sisters of operated women for SUI as compared to 40.3% among mothers and 11.6% among sisters of continent women. It suggests that heredity may play a significant role.

Impact of Incontinence on Quality of Woman's Life:

Urinary incontinence substantially compromises the overall quality of life of women. There is a great amount of fear and stress among the incontinent women for coping with embarrassment and restriction of daily activities induced by incontinence.

Physical Impact: In immobilized patients and those recovering from illness urinary incontinence leads to disturbed sleep. More than 50% incontinent women are bothered by night time voiding leading to disturbed sleep. More frequent urge incontinence episodes may increase the risk of falls among elderly in the bathrooms leading to nursing home admissions.

Psychological Impact: The psychological impact of urinary incontinence may not be directly proportionate to the severity of incontinence. It involves more than hygiene. Patients, whose activities are limited, find it difficult to speak about their condition. Many patients suffer silently with symptoms for years, believing treatment to be ineffective. It poses a threat to self-esteem. Fear of odor of urine is most common because of which incontinent women feel embarrassed and ashamed.

Social Impact: Women with urge or mixed incontinence often limit their social activities. The performance of daily activities that most people take for granted necessitates elaborate planning or simply becomes impossible because of incontinence. Traveling by public transport becomes very difficult, limiting options for shopping or visiting friends and family. Finding accessible public toilet (toilet mapping) can be a prime source of anxiety. Most of women avoid going to public places with unknown restrooms. It also affects their hobbies, vacation and attending church or temple. It is most bothersome during journey.

Incontinence also has an impact on family life. In one study, 324 sexually active women were surveyed and 24% reported incontinence during sexual activity. Thus, sexual relations are also affected. Usually urge incontinence is more bothersome than stress incontinence. Patients with urge incontinence finds urinary leaks to be of greater problem than do those with stress incontinence because urge incontinence is less predictable and large volume of urine leak occurs. Urge incontinence often occurs at night, resulting in loss of sleep and the need to change clothes and bedding. This indicates that there is reduced quality of life and increased coping behavior among women with urge and mixed incontinence.

Financial Impact: Urinary incontinence is a costly condition because of the use of absorbent products, laundry cost, urinary tract and skin infections and drugs needed to manage incontinence. Supplementary costs which are more difficult to quantify include caregivers' time and women's isolation due to negative social stigma and hygienic problem associated with it. The financial burden is further compounded by the poor mobility, coordination and vision problem common among elderly persons who are at risk for falls and other accidents as a result of urge incontinence.

Diagnosis of Urinary Incontinence:

Urinary incontinence is a complex condition that can result from multiple interacting causes, including physiological, behavioral, emotional, social and environmental factors. Its successful management is dependent on a thorough evaluation that accurately characterizes the type of incontinence, and if possible, identifies the underlying etiology. The assessment process includes history and physical examination, measurement of post void residual, voiding diary, laboratory and perineal pad test and if indicated a urodynamic evaluation.

History:

Diagnosis of UI can be made according to symptoms alone, without referring to a specialist or invasive processes. Symptom analysis can detect 81% cases of genuine stress urinary incontinence accurately.

Voiding Diary:

A three day voiding diary is a simple and practical method of obtaining information on UI. Approaching diagnosis through the evaluation of symptoms obviates the invasive and expensive procedures requiring specialist referral.

Home pad testing:

Pads can be used to evaluate objectively the amount of urine lost. This can be combined with history to evaluate incontinence.

Barrier to treatment seeking for women in India:

In India, women in their natural role as mothers, sisters, wives and daughters have been accepted as the principal providers of good health to their families and indirectly to the community. Yet when it comes to their own health, women in India receive low priority. Women consider most of their reproductive morbidities as 'normal' and a part of their destiny. They may not seek treatment or may not report their symptoms. Even If they perceive it to be abnormal, they may conceal it out of guilt or shame as they take it as a punishment to their past deeds (theory of *karma*).

There is often a low consultation rate for any morbidity related to private parts. Women usually feel shy to discuss their health problems with male health team members. Like other Indians, women here also have a fatalistic attitude and that of "ignorance is bliss" Other reason for non consultation is poverty, lack of financial independence, and "culture of silence" In general; there is a scarcity of female doctors and urologists in India. And even they are often too busy to patiently listen and understand the problems of women and provide the treatment.

In India, surgery of any kind is usually a dreaded proposition and people tend to avoid it as far as possible, probably because of which women continue to suffer and tolerate the symptoms of any sort before resorting to operation, if at all when the situation becomes unbearable. Women give low priority to their health. They tend to suffer silently without seeking health care until it reaches severity, because of their shyness, poverty and dependence on their husband. In many instances lack of education and information may limit women's understanding of the benefit of health services. Thus, education is an important determinant in the utilization of health services.

Thus, there is poor utilization of health services not only because services are inaccessible to poor women but also because they are culturally inappropriate to women's needs and expectations Moreover, as indicated above, various handicaps and compulsions in women's lives force them to develop a tolerant attitude and a "culture of silence" towards their reproductive health problems.

Treatment of urinary incontinence:

Treatment goals for incontinence management are the elimination of symptoms and improvement of the quality of life. For urge and mixed incontinence, two approaches are used: pharmacological and non-pharmacological. But the effectiveness of either treatment may take as long as four weeks to become apparent. For stress urinary incontinence, surgical, pharmacological and non-pharmacological therapies are used. Treatment ranges from minor life style changes to surgery.

Non pharmacological management:

Life style modification: It is targeted towards reducing or eliminating risk factors like reduction of intake of caffeine or other dietary irritants (such as acidic fruit juices, colas, coffee and tea), smoking cessation, weight reduction. . Constipation and straining during bowel movement increases pressure on the bladder. Regulation of bowel movements helps to prevent urinary incontinence.

Behavioral Therapy:

Behavioral intervention should be considered the first line of treatment for urinary incontinence for patients who are motivated enough to devote time and effort for behavioral therapy in order to avoid invasive procedures.

Behavioral therapy describes a group of treatments that are based on the idea that incontinent patient can be educated about the condition. Strategies are developed to conservatively minimize or eliminate the incontinence. It is sometimes erroneously equated with and reduced to the combination of fluid restriction and timed voiding. But actually it is a far richer therapy. In fact, one of the

Table 1

Comparison of different modes of treatment for Urinary incontinence

Variables	*Modes of Treatment*		
	Medicine	*Surgery*	*Behavior Therapy*
Consultation & need of Follow-up(no.)	Multiple contacts needed	Multiple contact needed	Only one contact needed
Specialist consultation required	Yes	Yes	No
Invasive investigations required	Yes	Yes	No
Side effects & Complications	Headache, dry mouth, nausea, vomiting, blurred vision, constipation	Injury to bladder, hematoma, infection, urine retention, fistula, recurrent stress incontinence, urge incontinence	None
Fear of surgery	No	Yes	No
Easy & Acceptable	No	No (fear of surgery)	Yes
Cost	Yes	Yes (Rs. 20,000 -30,000)	No
Success rate	50-60%	30-90%	50-90%
Relapse	Yes	25-50%	10-15%
Duration of treatment	Long	One time surgery	8-12 weeks daily exercise and then a habit is formed

main problems with the term "behavior therapy" is that it has been used so differently by practitioners that its meaning has become dilute and vague. There is no standard protocol or best methodology for behavior therapy of urinary incontinence. Behavioral therapy must start with instruction about normal urinary tract anatomy and function. Patient needs to understand the role of the bladder and pelvic floor muscles. A voiding diary is used to teach patient about his or her bladder function. This diary becomes a basis for evaluation and goal setting for desired voiding interval. Repeated evaluations are made in which patient's performance is compensated with goals and new goals are set, providing positive reinforcement. Patients are taught urge inhibition. Kegels exercises are a part of such therapy.

Bladder training: It is strongly recommended for the management of urge and mixed incontinence and also recommended for stress incontinence.

Pelvic floor muscle exercises: These are strongly recommended for women with stress urinary incontinence.

As the table 1 illustrates the utility of behavioral therapy can be realized when we compare it with the surgical and drug therapy for incontinence. Women with pure stress incontinence respond well to surgical therapy with cure rate of 35-95%. Women with urge incontinence benefit from drug intervention, with cure or improvement of 50-60%. However both drugs and surgery have side effects and risks are involved hence, behavior therapy should be considered as initial step for management of incontinence before considering surgical or medical intervention.

Impact of Behavior Therapy:-

A study conducted by the authors at PGIMER Chandigarh concluded that behavior therapy **intervention** led to a rapid and highly significant improvement in the severity of urinary incontinence in the study group. Out of total **mild** cases, **77% were fully cured** and rest had no leak episode since training. **71% of moderate cases were completely cured** and 16% changed into mild. Out of total **severe urinary incontinence cases 34% became continent** and 1/3rd became mild. At the end of follow-up, overall **52.5% women were continent and 24.4% became mild**. So, **77% cases** were benefited by intervention. Out of these cases 73%

respondents reported complete relief from incontinence immediately after the 8 weeks intervention phase (weekly session one contact) was over.

Limitation of behavior therapy is that it is most effective in mild and moderate cases of incontinence. Those who do not have improvement after 4-6 weeks should consult the doctor. But behavior therapy is safe and it could be continued along with medication and after surgery to prevent recurrence of problem.

Conclusion: Incontinence causes a lot of distress, embarrassment and inconvenience among the affected women. It remains one of the most common social and hygiene problems of women. Incontinent women need not suffer silently. They must be encouraged to seek help and to discuss their problems openly with their health care providers. Infact, most of the mild and moderate cases can be managed conservatively at the primary care level.

Training Module on Behaviour Therapy for Leakage of Urine Among Women

Involuntary loss/leakage of urine is called **Urinary Incontinence**. It is a significant social and hygienic health problem among women. It can vary from occasional botheration/problem of leaking a few drops of urine to a more serious problem of leaking ample amount of urine several times a day. It has severe economic and psychosocial impact on women's lives. It is a heavy emotional burden for women in terms of embarrassment, social isolation and diminished self-prestige. Such women are often not willing to seek help. Some view it as a routine part of their lives. Many do not report it as health problem to doctors because in Indian society it is not considered good to discuss women's illness with strangers.

Why leakage occurs: Leakage of urine occurs as **pelvic floor muscles** become weak with age and repeated childbirths. Moreover, hormonal changes associated with menopause also cause weakness of muscles leading to incontinence.

Affected women often feel embarrassed and ashamed. They go on suffering without telling anyone. If it is left untreated for long, it gets worse and operation may be needed.

But one should know that it is very simple to control and correct this defect without operation. This can be achieved through special exercises which all women can do easily. These exercise helps in strengthening **pelvic floor muscles**. This manual describes how women themselves can get rid of this problem by self-care.

Three types of urinary incontinence are there:

1.Stress urinary incontinence: It is sudden leakage of a small amount of urine. It usually occurs with coughing, sneezing, laughing, lifting weight, bending and standing from sitting position.

2.Urge incontinence: It is characterized by a strong desire to pass urine that occurs immediately prior to leakage of urine. Such individuals tell that they cannot reach the toilet on time and leakage occurs. Some may report frequent need to go for urination. Some even report passing urine in the bed during sleep.

3. Mixed incontinence: It refers to a combination of stress incontinence and urge incontinence symptoms.

HOW THE BLADDER WORKS

You must have observed small children passing urine in bed and even in clothes. They do so because in children, the bladder gradually fills with urine, the bladder expands and signals spinal cord that it is getting increasingly full. Bladder filling continues as it reaches a critical point, when spinal cord signals bladder to empty itself. This is called as voiding reflex.Our brain has no control over it.

At this stage urine control is without any connection to brain as it occurs in babies.

When a child is 2-3 yrs old we teach him where and when to pass urine. Slowly, over time, children learn to control urine and pass urine when they reach toilet.

To control when the bladder empties, person must learn to control voiding reflex . This learning takes place in early childhood.Through their parents/caretakers children learn to void when they reach toilet. Even if voiding reflex is there, it is the brain which controls continence and muscles help by keeping in them closed until you reach toilet. Continence is, therefore, a learned behaviour and habit.

But you must know, this training will help you to control your urine leakage problem. But it will not give instant result. As you will continue exercise you will notice improvement in 2-3 weeks. Be patient and continue with your exercises.

STRUCTURE OF URINARY SYSTEM

To understand the exercise therapy for cure of incontinence, it is important to understand the structure & functioning of urinary system especially the lower urinary tract in women.

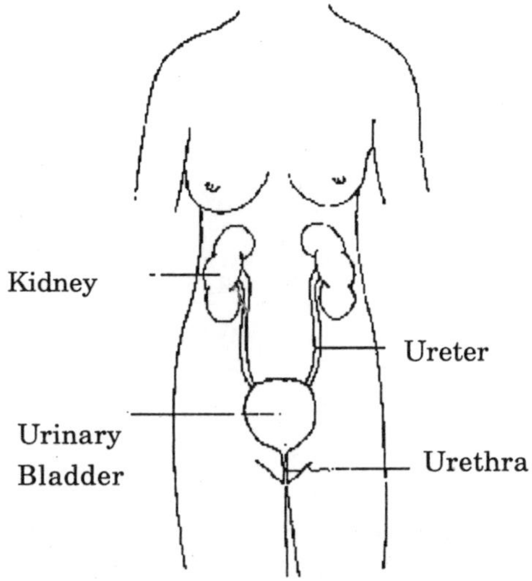

Fig. 1: Urinary System

The urinary system in human performs the task of collecting waste and removing them from body in the form of urine. It consists of two kidneys, two ureters, a urinary bladder and a urethra (Fig. 1).

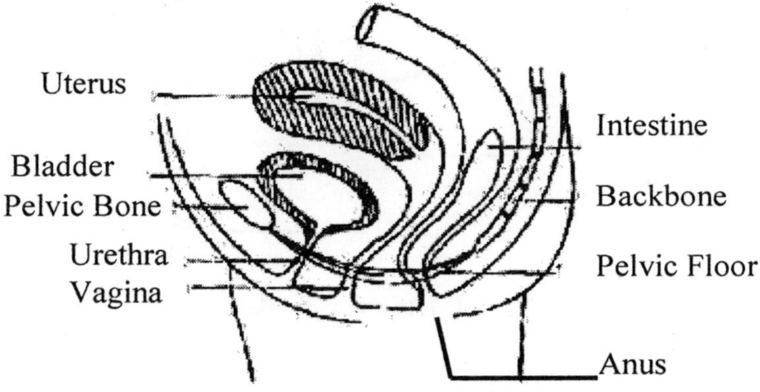

Fig. 2: View of the Pelvic Floor

Pelvic floor consists of muscles and connective tissue that stretches from tail bone to pubic bone like a sheet. These muscles and the connective tissue support the lower urinary tract organs (urinary bladder & urethra) as well as the uterus and rectum (Fig. 2, 3).

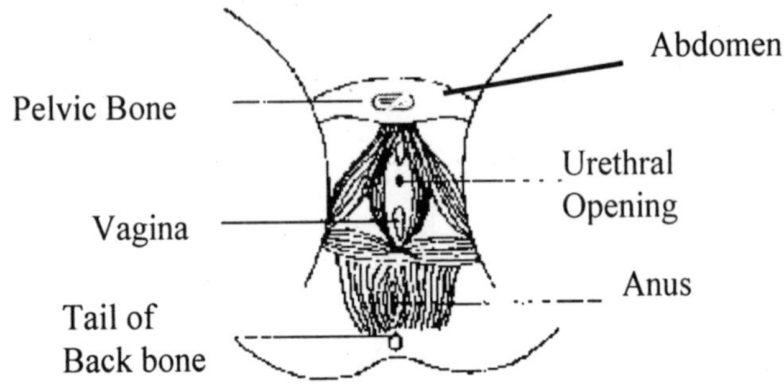

Fig. 3

The urinary bladder is a hollow bag like organ. It has muscles in its lining. When the bladder is full the urine is expelled through urethra by contraction of the bladder muscles (Fig. 4).

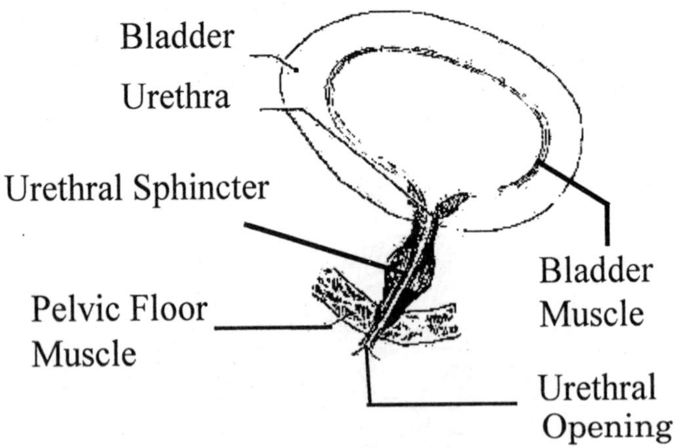

Fig. 4: Urinary System

Female urethra is a short tube about 3 to 4 cm (1 to 1.5 inch) in length consisting of layer muscles. It is encircled at middle part by the external **urethral sphincter**, a voluntarily controllable muscle (a kind of valve/lid/plug) which controls leakage of urine.

THERE ARE TWO PHASES IN URINATION

1.Storage Phase: (1) During this phase bladder fills gradually with urine which is formed in kidneys. (2) Bladder muscle remains inactive, although it expands passively to accommodate urine (Fig. 5, 6). Usually about 150-250 ml of urine can be stored before bladder pressure begins to rise and first desire to urinate is perceived. During this time sphincter increases its resistance and signal from brain allows bladder to fill further up to maximum capacity of 350-500 ml.

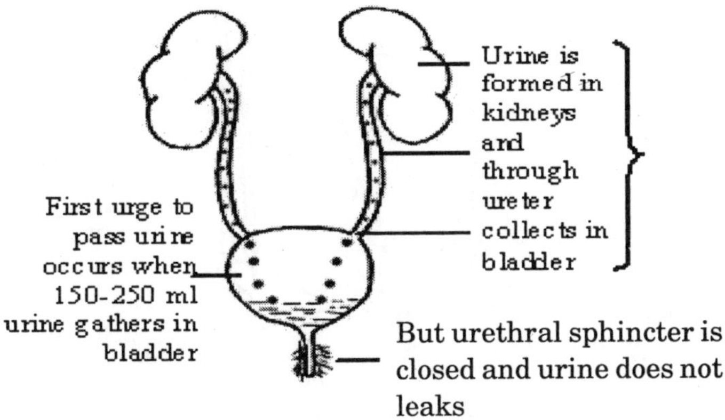

Fig. 5: Collection of Urine in Bladder

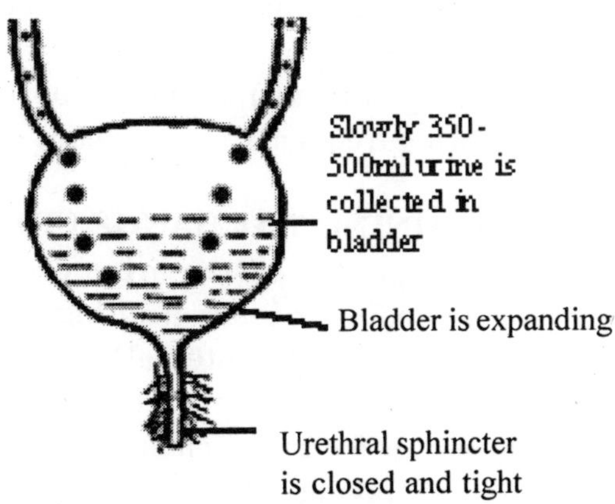

Fig. 6: Bladder is full with urine but urethral sphincter is closed

2.Expulsion Phase : When the bladder is full to its capacity signal goes to brain and getting OK from it, bladder muscle contracts pushing urine out of bladder and the bladder neck sphincter relaxes, allowing urine to pass through urethra (Fig. 7). It means passing urine is controlled by brain.

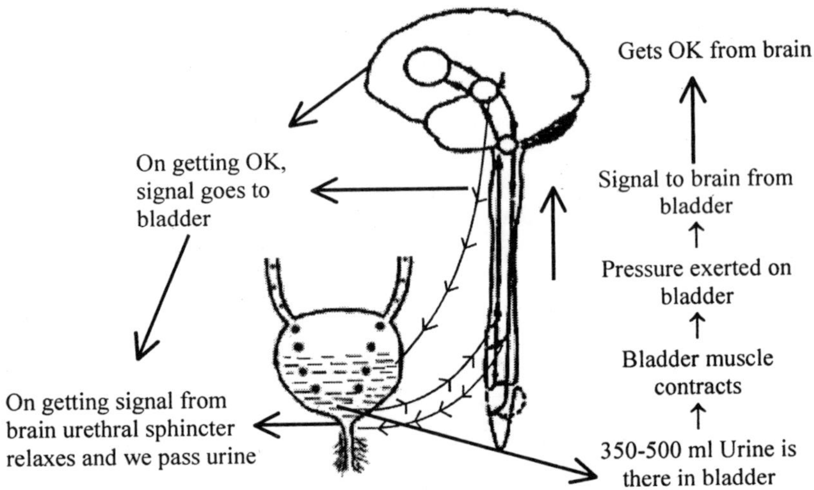

Fig. 7: Process Controlling the Urinary System by Brain

Normally, a person passes urine 5 to 7 times per 24 hours. Thus, there is a 3 to 4 hours interval between passing urine when we are awake. During night a person may go for urination before going to bed and then after getting up in the morning. Urination may be more frequent during winter and rainy season than in summer. Urination frequency also depends on liquid intake.

BLADDER TRAINING TO CHANGE URINATION HABIT

Normally a person passes urine every 3-4 hours.Bladder training involves finding an interval during which there is no leakage and gradually increasing this interval to a normal urination pattern of every 3-4 hours. Women who leak urine knowingly or unknowingly may go for urination more frequently than necessary. They believe that having less urine in the bladder decreases the chances of leakage. However, on the contrary, more frequent urination leads to development of a habit where brain sends a signal to go for urination even when less urine is there in bladder.

Usually, the first desire to urinate occurs when bladder is half full (150-250 ml). So when you get the first feeling to go for urination take deep breath and divert your attention from going to toilet. But if the urge is very strong you may go to toilet. Slowly, increase the interval between urination. Your target is to achieve an interval of 3-4 hours between urination within 6 weeks.

It is the **brain that controls your urination signal. Bladder muscles work according to the signal**. So it is important to correct your habit of frequently going to toilet by increasing the interval so that your bladder gets trained to hold normal amount of urine and your voiding interval of three to four hours is achieved. This can be facilitated by keeping a urination diary.

MYTH – More frequent urination prevents leakage.

REALITY – Rather, this leads to leakage of urine. Frequent urination sends wrong signals to brain.

WHAT TO DO – Do not pass urine frequently. Train your bladder to hold.

Actually rushing is the worst thing you can do.

- Rushing jiggles your bladder, increasing your awareness of how full it feels and making the urgency worse.
- Movement can stimulate the bladder to contract and empty.
- Rushing put extra-abdominal pressure on bladder and tends to push urine out.
- Rushing interferes with concentration that you need to control bladder.

Six simple steps to do when desire to urinate is felt.

1. Stop what you are doing, sit down when possible or stand quietly.
2. Contract your pelvic floor muscles quickly several times. Do not relax fully in between.
3. Take a few deep breaths.
4. Concentrate on suppressing the desire to urinate.
5. Wait until desire to urinate subsides.
6. Walk to bathroom at normal pace. Do not rush, continue contracting you pelvic floor muscles while you reach toilet.

Bladder training is like forming a habit, just like teaching a child to control his urination. So you have to learn to pass urine at regular interval. But be patient as results are not instant, Results will be noticeable offer 2-3 weeks. So be patient and continue your training.

HOW TO PREVENT URINE LEAKAGE

a) Lifestyle changes & dietary modifications for prevention of urine leakage

Leakage of urine can be prevented by changing our life style/ activities. Often a person with incontinence restricts the liquid intake thinking that it will prevent leakage. This practice is harmful. This not only reduces bladder capacity but also increases the risk of constipation and bladder irritation leading to leakage.

1. Increase fluid intake to 8-10 glasses per day i.e. 1.5 – 2 liter. This helps not only to dilute bladder irritants but also to increase bladder capacity. (Do not take too much liquid at one time but take it at equal and regular intervals). Sufficient water/liquids should be taken to satisfy your thirst.
   DO NOT RESTRICT FLUID INTAKE
2. Take fiber rich diet e.g. whole grains, fruits and vegetables and salads to relieve constipation. Constipation itself can precipitate incontinence. Constipation is a risk factor for leakage of urine.
   AVOID CONSTIPATION – AVOID LEAKAGE
3. Do not smoke as it can produce cough and exaggerate incontinence.
   SAY NO TO SMOKING AND STAY DRY
4. Always lift heavy objects with care or get help for lifting, if needed. Lifting weight increases intra-abdominal pressure leading to incontinence.
   BE CAREFUL WHILE LIFTING – AVOID LEAKAGE
5. If you are overweight, try to reduce your weight to normal.
   OBESITY IS A RISK FACTOR FOR LEAKAGE
6. Avoid irritable fluids such as tea, coffee and cold drinks. These fluids cause bladder irritation leading to leakage.
   TEA, COFFEE, COLD DRINKS LEAD TO – LEAKAGE
7. Avoid infection. Keep genital area/private part clean. Change and wash your undergarments daily. Wear cotton underwear. Maintain menstrual hygiene.
   INFECTION CAN LEAD TO URINE LEAKAGE
8. Avoid mental stress.

URINATION DIARY

To know your success with training, you are required to maintain urination diary. (Make a 24 hr diary).

Instructions

Please record each time you drink fluid, each time you pass urine in toilet or leak accidentally. Do this for three consecutive days.

- Whenever you drink water please ✓ in column 1.
- Whenever you drink tea, coffee, cold drink, milk, juice, lassi please ✓ in column 2.
- If normal urine is passed in toilet put ✓ in column 3.
- In the column of "urine leak" tick under column (o) for a drop or two, (O) for enough requiring you to change clothes or smell (in column 5).
- If you had sudden urge to void and you could not reach toilet in time. Tick P in column 4.
- In "activity" column 6 tick if leak occurred during (e.g. coughing, sneezing, laughing, lifting heavy objects, rising from chair, washing hands, hearing running water).

URINATION DIARY

Day 1 – Count from the time you got up from bed.

Time	*Fluid Intake*		*Normal Urination in Toilet*	*Urine Leak*			
	Water 1	*Cold drink Tea / Coffee* 2	3	*Could not reach toilet* 4	*Urine Leak* 5		*Activity when leak* 6
6 AM		200ml			o	O	Cough
7 AM							
8 AM							
9 AM							
10 AM							

PELVIC FLOOR MUSCLE EXERCISE (KEGEL'S EXERCISE)

These simple exercises can help in preventing leakage.

Basic information

Ø Pelvic floor muscle exercises can strengthen the muscle around vagina & increase your ability to contract & relax these muscles completely.

Ø Pelvic floor muscles are special in women because they support the organs in the pelvis (uterus, bowel & bladder). Keeping these muscles strong can help prevent urine leakage and even a uterine prolapse.

Ø With age, weakness develops in pelvic floor muscles due to normal wear & tear and child birth. The bladder, uterus & rectum begin to slip down and get squeezed into lower region of pelvis. Women can develop stress incontinence, urge incontinence or both. Performing exercises can help to prevent and relieve these symptoms.

TIPS FOR PRACTICING PELVIC FLOOR MUSCLE EXERCISE

How to identify correct muscle which needs to be exercised?

- To get the feel of the muscle alternatively start and stop urinating while using the toilet by tightening the muscle. If you can slow the stream of urine, even slightly, you are using the right muscle.

OR

- When you have urge to pass flatus in a gathering but you hold back the flatus by squeezing muscles around your anus; so that is the muscle we are talking about.

OR

- To find the muscle, place your finger inside your vagina or rectum and try to press your finger by contracting internal muscles. This is the muscle you have to exercise. This muscle is the same one you use to hold back gas or bowel movement.

Practicing the exercise

- Squeeze the muscle you have identified earlier for counts of ten (or ten seconds) then relax for ten seconds. Remember that, it is just as important to relax as it is to contract the muscle. Initially, you may not be able to hold this muscle for ten seconds. However, slowly over a period of two weeks you will be able to hold for ten seconds. Start with 3 seconds and over a period of 2-3 weeks increase it upto 10 seconds.

- Practice the tightening and relaxation while sitting, standing, walking and watching T.V. and even lying down. While lying down on your back with knees bent and feet 12 inch apart, arms resting on your side you can perform the exercise. Start with five times each and gradually work up to ten and then up to twenty times each time.
- Give a gap of 2 minutes after 5-6 contractions.
- Do fifteen exercise in the morning, fifteen in the afternoon and twenty at night or do the exercise for ten minutes 3 times a day or you can try to work up to twenty five exercises twice a day.
- In time, you will learn to practice effortlessly. Eventually, you will be able to work these exercises in as part of your lifestyle like brushing your teeth or eating a meal.
- If you leak urine when you cough or sneeze or laugh you should squeeze the muscle before coughing or sneezing or laughing. Once the muscle become strong and has some endurance you will have lesser amount/episodes of leakage. Do the pelvic muscle contractions whenever you anticipate extra pressure on your pelvis.
- **Remember:-** Never use your stomach, leg or buttock muscles for exercise. The most common mistake is to use too many muscles. To find out if you are also contracting your stomach muscles, place your hand on your abdomen while you squeeze your pelvic floor muscle. If you feel your abdomen move, then you are wrongly using these muscles. If so, you must change your technique.
- This exercise can be practiced any time, in any place. Since this muscle is internal, no one can notice you exercising this muscle.
- Build strength slowly. Do not expect results right away. You can notice a little bit of change after two weeks and by six weeks, benefits will be visible.

Do not hold breath while doing exercise, take normal breath.

Can these exercises harm me?

No, these exercises can not harm you in any way. Most patients find them relaxing and easy. If you have stomach pain or back pain after you exercise, then you are probably trying too hard or using stomach and back muscles. If so, again try to find the correct muscles. Remember, exercise should feel mild and easy. Do not exercise under tension. Remember to focus on relaxation as well as squeezing the muscle. When you will learn to practice effortlessly the exercises can be a part of your lifestyle like brushing teeth or eating a meal. This will help you to remain OK for a lifetime and there will never be a urine leakage problem.

You may be tempted to stop exercising your pelvic floor muscles. But remember! you have worked hard to strengthen these muscles. If you stop exercising, now, they will weaken again. So only way to maintain strength of your muscles is to keep exercising them regularly. This was you will remain continent and leaking will not occur.

How to maintain record of your exercise: You are provided with a form where you will

- Tick mark three times if you are exercising three times daily.
- Tick mark two times if you are exercising two times daily.
- Tick mark one times if you are exercising once daily.
- Put cross mark if you are not exercising.

Day	*Date*	*Exercise*		
		Sitting	*Lying Down*	*Standing*
1				
2				
3				
4				
5				
6				
7				
8				
9				

References

1. Rowe J.W., Besdine R.W., Ford A.B., Gartley C.B., Consensus Conference, Urinary Incontinence in Adults. JAMA 1989; 261: 2685-90.
2. Sampselle C.M. Behavioral intervention in young and middle age women; American Journal of Nursing. (Supplement).2003; 103: 9-19.
3. Mittal.N, Hota.D, Urinary Incontinence, Drugs Bulletin. 2008; 31: 1-16
4. Morkved S., Urinary incontinence during pregnancy and after delivery, effect of pelvic floor muscle training in prevention and treatment PhD Thesis, Norwegian University of Science and Technology 2003
5. Thakar R., Stanon S., Management of urinary incontinence in women. British Medical Journal, 2000; 321: 1326-30.
6. Resnick NM, Yalla SV. Management of urinary incontinence in the elderly. The New England Journal of Medicine, 1985; 113: 800-805.
7. Newman D.K., Giovannini. D. The overactive bladder: A nursing perspective". Am J of Nursing, 2002; 102: 36-45.
8. Bump R.C., Norton P.A. Epidemiology and natural history of pelvic floor dysfunction. Obstetrics and Gynecology Clinics of North America 1998; 25: 723-740.
9. Brown J.S. Epidemiology and changing demographies of overactive bladder: a focus on the postmenopausal women. Geriatrics 2003 Supplement 1; 57: 6-12.
10. Haillot P.O., Bruyere F., Boutin I.M., Bertrang P., Lanson Y. Prevalence and risk factors of urinary incontinence in young and middle-aged women. British Journal Urology International 2002; 89: 61-66
11. Skoner M., Thompson W.D., Caron V.A. Factors associated with risk of stress urinary incontinence in women. Nursing Research 1994; 43: 301-6
12. Kumari.S, Impact of a behavioral training package on occurrence and severity of urinary incontinence, Ph.D thesis, P.G.I.M.E.R. Chandigarh(2007)
13. Samuelsson E., Victor A., Svardsudd K. Determinants of urinary incontinence in a population of young and middle-aged women". Acta Obstet Gynecol Scand, 2000; 79: 1208-15

14. Hampel C., Wienhol D., Banken N., Eggersmann, C., Thuroff J.W. Prevalence and natural history of female incontinence. Eur. Urol. 1997; 32 (Suppl. 2): 3-12.
15. Henriette.J.Brummen.V. ummen.V. Bruinse.H.W, Pol.G.V.D, Peter.A.,Heintz.M, Huub.S, Vaart. V, Bothersome lower urinary tract symptoms 1 year after first delivery. Prevalence and the effect of child birth. British Journal of Urology International 2006; 98: 89-95.
16. Buchsbaum G.M., Chin M., Glantz C., Guzick D. Prevalence of urinary incontinence and associated risk factors in a cohart of nuns. Obstet Gynecol 2002; 100: 226-229.
17. Maclennan A.H., Taylor A.W., Wilson D.H., Wilson D. The prevalence of pelvic floor disorders and their relationship to gender, age, parity and made of delivery. British Journal of Obstetric and Gynecology 2000; 107: 1460-70
18. Lukaaz E.S., Lawrence J.M., Cantreras R., Nager C.W., Luber K.M. Parity, mode of delivery and pelvic floor disorders. Obstet Gynecol 2006; 107: 1253-66.
19. Sharma S., Walia I., Singh A. A case control study on uterine prolapse in a Chandigarh Slum. Bulletin PGIMER, 2003; 37: 143-48
20. Smith A.R.B., Hosker G.L., Warrell D.W. The role of partial denervation of the pelvic floor in the aetiology of genitourinary prolapse and stress urinary incontinence of urine. A neurophysiological study. British Journal of Obstetric and Gynecology, 1989; 96: 24-28.
21. Viktrup L., Lose G. The risk of stress incontinence 5 years after first delivery. Am J Obstet Gynecol 2001; 185: 82-87
22. Brown J.S., Grady D., Ouslander J.G., Herzog A.R., Varner R.E., Posner S.F. Prevalence of urinary incontinence and associated risk factors in postmenopausal women. Obstet Gynecol 1999; 94: 66-70.
23. Snooks S.J., Setchell M., Swash M., Henry M.M. Injury to innervation of pelvic floor sphincter musculature in child birth. The Lancet 1984; 334 ; 546-50.
24. Hvidman L., Fddsprung A., Mommsen S., Nelsen J.B. Postpartum urinary incontinence. Acta Obstet Gynecol Scand 2001; 82: 556-63.
25. MacArthur C., Glazener C,, Don Wilson P., Lancashire R.J., Herbison G.P., Grant A.M. Persistent urinary incontinence and delivery mode, history : a six year longitudinal study. Br J Obst Gynecology 2006; 113:1218-224
26. Viktrup L., Lose G. The risk of stress incontinence 5 years after first delivery. Am J Obstet Gynecol 2001; 185: 82-87

27. Fischer J.R., Berg P.H. Urinary incontinence in United States air force female aircrew. Obstet Gynecol 1999; 94: 532-36
28. Chaliha C., Kalia V., Stanton S.L., Monga A., Sultan A.H. Antenatal prediction of postpartum urinary & fecal incontinence. Obstet. Gynecol 1999; 94: 689-94
29. Viktrup L., Lose G., Rolff M., Barfoed K. Symptoms of stress incontinence caused by pregnancy or delivery in primiparas. Obstet. Gynecol. 1992; 79: 945-49.
30. Bo K., Stien R., Hansen S.K., Kristofferson M. Clinical and urodynamic assessment of nulliparous young women with and without stress incontinence symptoms: A case control study. Obstet. Gynecol. 1994; 84: 1028-32.
31. Nygaard I.E., Thompson F.L., Sarah A.T.C., Svengalis L., Albright J.P. Urinary incontinence in Elite Nulliparous Athletes. Obstet Gynecol 1994; 84: 183-7.
32. Hannestad Y.S., Rortvert G., Dattveit A.K., Hunskaar S. Are smoking and other life style factors associated with female urinary incontinence? The Norwegian Epincont Study. British Journal of Obstet Gynecology, 2003; 110: 247-54.
33. Bump R.C., McClish D.M. Cigarette smoking and pure genuine stress incontinence of urine: A comparison of risk factors and determinants between smokers and non-smokers. Obstet Gynecol 1994; 170: 579-82.
34. Hannestad Y.S., Rortveit G., Sandvik H., Hunskaar S. A community-based epidemiological survey of female urinary incontinence: The Norwegian Epincont Study. Journal of Clinical Epidemiology 2000; 53: 1150-57.
35. Grodstein F., Lifford K., Resnick N.M., Curhan G.C. Post menopausal Haemon therapy and risk of developing urinary incontinence. Obstet Gynecol 2004; 103: 254-60.
36. Arya L.A., Myers D., Jackson N. Dietary caffeine intake and the risk for detrusor instability: A case control study. Obstet Gynecol 2000; 96: 85-87.
37. Ertunc D, Tok EC, Pata O, Dilek U, Ozdemir G, Dilek S. Is stress urinary incontinence a familial condition? Acta Obstet. Gynecol Scand 2004; 83: 912-16.
38. Singh A, Arora A.K. Effect of uterine prolapse on the lives of rural north Indian women. Singapore Journal of Obstetric and Gynecology.2003; 34:52-58.

39. Kumari. S, Walia I.J. and Singh A.J. Self reported uterine prolapse in a resettlement colony of North India. Journal of Midwifery and Women's Health.2000; 45: 343-350.
40. Wyman J.F., Harkins Stephen W., Choi S.C., Taylor J.R., Fantl JA. Psychosocial impact of urinary incontinence in women. Obstet Gynecol 1987; 70: 378-81.
41. Dubeau C.E. The continuum of urinary incontinence in an aging population. Geriatrics, 2003 (Supplement) 1; 57: 12-17
42. Hilton P., Urinary incontinence during sexual intercourse: A common, but rarely volunteered symptom. British Journal of Obstetrics & Gynecology 1988; 95: 377-381.
43. Wilson L., Brown J.S., Shin G.P., Luc K., Subak L. Annual direct cost of urinary incontinence. Obstet Gynecol, 2001; 98: 398-406.
44. Versi E., Cardozo L., Anand D., Cooper D. Symptoms analysis for the diagnosis of genuine stress incontinence. Br J of Obstetric and Gynecology, 1991; 98: 815-19.
45. Fink. D, Perucchin. D, Schaer. G.N, Haller. V, The role of the frequency volume chart in the differential diagnosis of female urinary incontinence. Acta Obstet-Gynecol Scand, 1999; 78: 254-57
46. Hawkins J., Gordone B. Shaw's Textbook of Gynecology, Padubidri. V.G., Daftary, S.N., (Editors) New Delhi. Elsevier India Pvt. Ltd., 13th edition: 187-193.
47. Davila G.W, Gurette N. Current treatment options for female urinary incontinence – A review. Int J Fertility 2004; 49: 102-12.
48. Fant J.A., Wyman J.F., Anderson R., Matt D., Bump R.C. Postmenopausal urinary incontinence: Comparison between non-estrogen supplemented and estrogen supplemented women. Obstet Gynecol, 1988; 71: 823-28.
49. Dmochowski R., Miklus J.R., Norton P., Zinner N., Yalein I., Bump R.C., Duloxetine versus placebo for the treatment of North American women with stress urinary incontinence. J Urology, 2003; 170: 1259-63.
50. Peattie A.B., Plevnik S., Stanon S.L. Vaginal cones: a conservative method of treating stress continence. Br Journal of Obstetric and Gynecology, 1988; 95: 1049-53.
51. Payne C.K. Behavioral therapy for overactive bladder. Urology 2000; 55 (Supple 5A): 3-6.
52. Burgio K.L., Pearce K.L., Lucco A.J., Staying Dry. A Practical Guide to Bladder Control. 1989 Baltimore, John Hopkins University Press: 1-120.

53. Fantl J.A., Wyman J.F., Mcclish D.K., Harkins S.W., Elswick R.K., Taylor J.R., Hadley E.C. Efficacy of bladder training in order women with urinary incontinence. JAMA 1991, 265: 609-13.
54. Kumari S, Jain V, Mandal A.K. and Singh A.J. Behaviour therapy for urinary incontinence in Indian Women. International Journal of Obstetrics & Gynecology. 2008; 103:125-130.
55. Kumari S, Jain V and Singh A.J. Treatment seeking behaviour for urinary incontinence in north Indian Women. Indian Journal of Medical Sciences. 2008; 62:352-356.

39

Vaginal discharge: Effect of Sitz Bath

Ranjit Kaur, Neelam Aggarwal, Avinash Kaur Rana and Sushma Kumari Saini

'With regard to vaginal discharge, women often receive little or no information regarding its genesis, how it is transmitted, how it can be treated, or how it can be prevented. Most affected women are convinced that vaginal discharge is a natural part of being a woman, and that they are condemned to suffer from it for life, particularly if they maintain an active sexual life'. (Leda Pesce)

Vaginitis among women of child bearing age is a common gynecological problem, often ignored and untreated, especially among women living in rural and urban slums. India is a poverty ridden country. Health problems of women are still largely ignored. Moreover women still consider it a taboo not to discuss their gynecological problems like vaginitis. Women are reluctant to seek medical treatment in India because of lack of privacy, lack of a female doctor at the health facility, cost of treatment and their subordinate social status. This reluctance is exacerbated when symptoms are embarrassing, as they are with Reproductives Tract Infections (RTI), especially among women of child bearing age groups. A "culture of silence" shrouds gynecologic morbidity throughout India and developed countries. They regard it as normal discomfort and therefore often do not seek medical treatment.

Reproductive Tract Infections (RTI), which are preventable and treatable, are responsible for causing serious consequences of infertility, ectopic pregnancy, pregnancy wastage, low birth weight babies etc. In a community based study in India, among the RTIs the range as evidenced by various studies is: cervicitis (21-86%), Pelvic inflammatory disease (19-45%) and Vaginitis (21-32%). As reproductive Tract Infections are the infections of the genital tract, they affect both women and men. Some RTIs (such as syphilis and gonorrhoea) are sexually transmitted but many are not.

Causes of RTI may be due to overgrowth of endogenous microorganisms normally found in the vagina. Endogenous organisms from the vagina or sexually transmitted organisms in the cervix may be pushed into the upper genital tract and cause serious infection of the uterus, tubes and other pelvic organs. Organisms from outside the body can also be introduced into the upper genital tract during medical procedures including insertion of copper T and induced abortions particularly if infection control is poor.[5] In women, RTIs can be asymptomatic and even when they are symptomatic their presentation can overlap with and be misdiagnosed as normal physiological change. Many times normal physiologic discharge may be misdiagnosed as RTI.

Vaginitis may have one or more of the following causes: bacterial or fungal infection; intestinal worms; vitamin B deficiency; congestion of the pelvic organs; gonococci; chemical irritation (strong douches); mechanical irritation (tampons); drug medications and deodorant sprays.

Other contributing factors include tight and nonporous clothing, diabetes, use of antibiotics, Vitamin-B_6 deficiency due to use of birth control pills and changes in the vaginal pH. Pregnancy increases the vaginal pH and also its glycogen content which is favorable to yeast infection. Tight-fitting synthetic underwear provides poor ventilation and a warm-moist environment for yeast infection to occur. Excess sugar and refined carbohydrates also help in feeding yeast infection. Normally the pH of the vagina is acidic anything that alkalinizes it contributes to vaginitis. The most common after effect of antibiotic therapy in women is a vaginal yeast infection. Frequent douching upsets vaginal pH and flora. Excessive intercourse, without proper lubrication, irritates vaginal walls. About 5% of women, who are given antibiotics for acne, develop vaginitis. Copper T produces a favorable environment for yeast infection, since they reduce normal vaginal secretions.

The composition of vaginal flora changes with age, stress, hormonal influence and sexual activity. Vaginitis is a diagnosis based on the presence of symptoms of abnormal discharge, vulvovaginal discomfort or both. Discharge flows from the vagina daily as the body's way of maintaining environment. Normal discharge is usually clear or milky with no bad odor. A change in the amount, irritation, itching or burning could be due to an imbalance of healthy bacteria in the vagina.

The overgrowth of normally present bacteria and infecting bacteria causes symptoms of vaginitis. Chemical irritation can also be a significant factor. Atrophic vaginitis includes symptoms like: dyspareunia, dryness, pruritus and abnormal bleeding. Bacterial vaginosis accounts for 40-50% of vaginitis cases, 20-25% of candidiasis, and 15-20 % of trichomoniasis.

Vaginitis is very commonly manifested with vaginal discharge, which is abnormal in colour, odour or amount. Pruritis, genital swelling, dysuria or lower abdominal or back pain may accompany the discharge. It is the common gynecological complaint of sexually active women and the causative organisms are Trichomonas, Candida and combination of Gardnerella and vaginal anaerobes. It is commonly called Leucorrhoea in scientific terms or "*Safed pani*" in layman's language.[10] Bacterial Vaginosis may be merely an acute or episodic condition, may become persistent, or may resolve spontaneously. The most common etiologies in adults resulting in symptoms of vaginitis include Candidiasis, Trichomonas vaginalis, and bacterial vaginosis.[8]

Candidiasis is a fungal infection common in women of child bearing age that results in thick, white vaginal discharge. Candidiasis is usually not contracted from a sexual partner. Seventy-five percent of ladies have episodes of candidiasis in their life time and recurrent episodes may indicate underlying disease of diabetes.

Trichomoniasis is associated with risk factors for other sexually transmitted diseases and with history of multiple sexual partners. The discharge is usually copious and frothy. Pruritus may be present. Symptoms often peak just after menses. Trichomoniasis is the most common non viral STD in the world. Infection during pregnancy has been resulting in preterm deliveries and low birth weight. [14].

Bacterial vaginosis is asymptomatic in up to 50% of women. If a discharge is present it will be homogenous grayish white or yellowish white. Bacterial vaginosis is common in pregnancy associated with preterm birth.

In India, community-based studies on the prevalence of RTI among women have been few but all of them have revealed a very high prevalence rate, ranging from 19 to as high as 86 per cent. A study conducted (1992) at a resettlement colony at a Chandigarh revealed that 21.6 % females had vaginal discharge. Another study was conducted in Chandigarh (1995), which reported that 61.5% married women reported one or two symptoms. Vaginal discharge was reported by 18.2% of females. Recently a study conducted (2004) in resettled colony of Chandigarh reported that 13.9% of the females have faced excessive vaginal discharge for a duration ranging from 1 month to 8 years. Vaginitis very often goes unattended or untreated, especially if women are living in rural areas and are poor and illiterate. Sometimes it is of acute nature and most of the times it becomes chronic in nature.

Most of the women suffer from one or more gynecological problems throughout their life. Among these leucorrhoea or vaginal discharge causing vaginitis is a common problem seen in every day gynecological practice. Still its inadequate treatment is one of the most difficult problems. This leads to high maternal morbidity in their reproductive life. Often attention is drawn to the symptom when the discharge is sufficient to cause burning and itching or soil the clothing, so that a pad is required.

India is a poverty ridden country and diagnostic investigations for RTIs are costly and beyond the reach of the common public. The rural areas are worst affected due to dearth of simple, inexpensive and reliable diagnostic tools for this recalcitrant problem. Many women consider most reproductive morbidities to be normal and a part of their destiny and may not report the symptoms / conditions to the health worker in a community setting.

WHO has recommended a syndromic management of reproductive tract infections which is based on symptoms and clinical signs. According to this approach a health worker at the most peripheral level in the community can diagnose these infections and accordingly give intervention or advise referral of the patient.

Diagnosis of a presumed STIs/RTIs has traditionally been based on either clinical diagnosis, which is often inaccurate or incomplete laboratory diagnosis which is complex, very expensive and may delay treatment. As early as the 1970s, public health physicians, particularly working in Africa, became interested in testing simple clinical tools for controlling and treating RTIs and STIs. This resulted in the design and promotion of "syndromic management" guidelines by the WHO in 1991.

Commonly prescribed medications do not only kill off some of the bad bacteria but may also wipe out all the good ones which are critical to keep vaginal immune system healthy. In the end medications tend to weaken the entire system and destroy the good vaginal flora causing recurrent infections.

Oral antifungal agents are highly effective for treating a single episode of thrush (vaginitis). Anti-fungal drugs can be administered orally or vaginally for the treatment of candidiasis.[59] About 1 in 10 women who experience an episode of thrush can go on to develop recurrent candidiasis.

Various studies were conducted showing the treatment of vaginitis with Sitz Bath. Various recommendations have been reported for the treatment of vaginitis with different forms of Sitz Bath like; Saline Sitz Bath, warm water Sitz Bath, Sitz Bath with baking soda, cold Sitz Bath, thick salt water Sitz Bath, diluted vinegar water Sitz Bath, soda water Sitz Bath etc.

A sitz bath (hip bath) is a type of bath in which only hips and buttocks are soaked in water or saline solution. The water may contain medication. 'Sitz' comes from the German verb "sitzen" meaning "to sit". A sitz bath is used for patients to ease the pains of hemorrhoids, uterine cramps, and painful ovaries. It is also used to ease discomfort from infection of the bladder or vagina. Vaginitis is also commonly treated as a supportive therapy with sitz bath. The cause of the infection determines the appropriate treatment. It may include oral or topical antibiotics or antifungal creams or similar medications. Treatment focuses on improved hygiene and Sitz Bath.

Many studies have been conducted on effect of salt (saline) water Sitz Bath in comparison with diluted vinegar water Sitz Bath in the treatment of vaginitis. The clinical effects of both treatment methods were 100% after one week of treatment. Salty water changes the pH of the vagina and makes it acidic in nature and it also helps in reducing the itching of the vaginal cavity. Sitz bath is also recommended often to soothe pain. Since in reproductive age group the ladies are more prone to have vaginitis, sitz bath is simple home based intervention for the treatment of vaginitis.

PROCEDURE OF SITZ BATH

ARTICLES :

(a) Basin / Tub
(b) Common Salt
(c) A teaspoon
(d) Container with warm water

PROCEDURE :

1. Explain the procedure to the client and take verbal consent.
2. Instruct the client to contract and relax pelvic floor muscles while taking Sitz Bath.
3. Maintain privacy.
4. Ensure that the client has emptied her bladder.
5. Wash hands and collect all articles.
6. Fill the basin/ tub with five liters of warm water in the bathroom. (1/2 of the basin should be filled with water)
7. Check the temperature of the water by putting it on dorsal surface of the hand.
8. Add 50 grams of salt in 5 liters of warm water.
9. Assist the client to remove her *salwar* and under garments.
10. Make the client sit in the basin with buttocks immersed in warm water, keeping her legs and feet out of the basin for 20 mins.
11. After completion of 20 mins, assist the client in drying and putting on her dress.
12. Wash hands.
13. Document the procedure.

Evidence

A study was conducted by National Institute of Nursing Education, PGIMER, and Chandigarh in Dhanas village near Chandigarh which is a rural setting. Among rural women 12.3% were found to have at least two symptoms of vaginitis and vaginal smiar showed positive growth of bacteria Sitz bath with salt water was administered to selected 40 subjects for 20 minutes duration for five days and on 6th day, their vaginal smear was checked again to assess the effect of intervention on the study population. It was seen that there was significant improvement in the laboratory report as well as in symptoms of vaginitis. Hence, home base management for the relief of the symptoms of vaginitis with saline sitz bath can be a viable option for affected women.

References

1. Bang RA, Bang AT, Baitule M, Chaudhary Y, Sarmukaddam S, Tale O. High prevalence of gynaecological disease in rural Indian women. The Lancet 1989; 1: 85-8.
2. World Health Organization (WHO), global Prevalence and incidence of selected curable sexually transmitted infections: Overview and estimates, Genava: WHO, 2001.
3. Baljit K. Kaistha KC. Prevalence of reproductive morbidities in young females of a resettled slum population. Nursing & midwifery Research Journal 2004; 11: 1-8.
4. Paxton LA. Kijwwanuka N. Natugoda F. Community based study of treatment seeking among subjects with symptoms of sexually transmitted diseases in rural Uganda .BMJ 1998; 317:1630-1.
5. Wilson C. Recurrent vulvo vaginitis candidiasis, an overview of traditional and alternative therapies Adv Nurse Precet 2005; 13 (5): 24-.
6. Garg S, Khokar A, Singh MM, Mehra M (2001). Utilization of Health Care Services for RTIs by dwellers of an urban slum of Delhi. Souvenier of Indian Public Health Congress, April 14-16 (Abstracts).
7. Gupta P, Ramachandaran VG, Sharma P, Talwar P (2000). Prevalence of RTI in women of a resettlement are of east Delhi. Souvenier of India Public Health Congress, April 14-16 (Abstract).
8. Walter E. Diagnosis of chlamydia trachomatis genitourinary infection. Annals of internal medicine 1988; 108:710-717.
9. Palai P. Singh A. Treating Vaginal discharge in slim women. Bull PGI 1944; 28:107-110.
10. Bang RA. High Prevalence of Gynecological Diseases in Rural Indian women. The lancet 1989: 85-88.

11. World Health organization. Guidelines for the management of sexually transmitted infections. Geneva: WHO, WHO / HIV AIDS/ 2001:01
12. Nyirjesy, P, Weitz MV, Grody MH, Lorber B. Over-the-counter and alternative medicines in the treatment of chronic vaginal symptoms. Obstetrics & Gynecology 1999;90:50-2.
13. Amsel, Totten PA, Spiegel CA, et al. Nonspecific vaginitis: Diagnostic Criteria and Microbial and Epidemiological Associations. Am J Med 1983; 74: 14-22.
14. Chatterjee J. Walia I.J. and Singh, A.J., (1995). Case control study on vaginal discharge. Indian Medical Gazette 129: 66-71.
15. Parvez S, Walia I, Dhaliwal L.K. and Singh, A.J. (1995). Vaginal discharge cases in a slum. Bull PGI, 29: 72-74.
16. Singh AJ. Vaginal discharge - Its causes and associated symptoms as perceived by rural north Indian Women. Indian Journal of Community Medicine, 2007; 32: 22-26.
17. Kaur Ranjit, Aggarwal Neelam, Rana Avinash Kaur. A quasi experimental study on sitz bath and its effect on vaginitis among women of reproductive age group residing at rural community hanas, Chandigarh. An unpublished thesis of National Institute of Nursing Education, PGIMER, Chandigarh submitted to Punjab University Chandigarh 2007.

40

Yoga for Women

Mohinder Singh

Introduction :- Yoga for women is helpful at every stage of life. Yogic exercises make women aware of their strengths and weakness while reducing stress, increasing flexibility and improving coordination etc. It is a good for their heart, respiratory and circulatory system. The practice of yoga also brings about suppleness of the spine and joints, stimulation of the glands, relaxation of the nervous centres and improvement of the digestive and eliminative powers of the body through various *asanas* and *pranayamas.*

How Yoga Works: Nowadays, society, suffers from strain, tension and maladies resulting from the exhausting demands of modern life. In such a scenario an ability to completely relax at will is an important asset. Every woman wants to look and feel good. She tries her best to be pretty and attractive and to enjoy life to the full. Yoga helps them to achieve all this. It helps them to improve their vitality, mental powers, sex impulses, beauty of face and figure. It helps them retain a youthful appearance as long as possible. Yogic exercises and techniques can also delay the menopause through its effect on the glands. It has been reported that yoga can restore menstruation in aging women. It feeds facial tissue and skin which become lined and wrinkled as these are starved of blood with aging because of poor blood with aging circulation. Practice of *Yoga Nidra* refreshes the nervous system and recharges the body. Breathing exercises of yoga preserve the vital energy. A series of *asanas* makes spine and body flexible through which all nerve impulses are sent to the brain. Mastery of relaxation techniques for completely resting muscles, nerves and mind is essential in retaining a youthful appearance.

At menarche, many young girls entering into physical maturity have trouble with menstruation. Sometimes these are periods do not the appear, sometimes, these are painful and profuse. Menstrual troubles are not only trials of adolescence many; girls become overweight, their complexion become blotchy and faces are often disfigured with pimples and acne. In this also, yoga can help the growing girls.

Pregnancy :- There are many yogic exercises which can facilitate natural childbirth. Expectant mothers can do breathing exercises, forward stretching and all the cross legged positions. Special emphasis is given on breathing and relaxation.

Menopause: Sooner or later, every woman must go through the menopause when her period of childbearing and menstruation comes to an end. Often, there are hot flushes, giddiness, palpitation, insomnia, depression, irritability. In addition there may be psychological fears and anxieties. The result is often extreme suffering sometime causing complete lack of balance and even insanity. Middle – age women often face problems like lack of interest, mood swings and lack of sleep all due to hormonal imbalance.

Daily Practice of shavasana and deep breathing will help to combat insomnia and nervous anxiety in menopausal women. Yoga can also help reduce the tension that so often finds expression in emotional outburst.

Asanas for menopause:

- Shavasana
- Shoulder stand posture (sarvang asana)
- Half shoulder stand posture (vipreet Karnimudra)
- Hal asana (Plough posture)

Women going through the menopause should have their B.P. checked regularly. Practice of shavasana will help reduce it.

For menstrual disorders following asanas may help

- Dhanur asana
- Bhujang asana

- Sarvang asana
- Matsya asana
- Hal asana
- Shalbh asana
- Anulom vilom pranayama
- Yog Nidra
- Pawanmuktasana 1 & 2

For obesity:- all above asanas, maha bandh and apana mudra are very effective

Diet :- Exercises are a great help in keeping as slim and well. But exercises alone cannot work miracles if people persist in taking a wrong diet and in over eating. Even the exercises which are otherwise effective will not really slim down a woman who regularly fills herself up with cakes, sweets, starches, drugs and alcohol. So alongwith yoga, diet should also be given due attention.

What we eat and how we eat it intimately affects our health and our looks. So, one should eat sensibly. One should keep one day fast in a week to keep the body system healthy.

Other measures should also be taken.

- Drink adequate amount of water
- Add fruits and fresh vegetables in your diet
- Stay happy and have positive attitude towards life

By following the above said tips it is possible enhance the effect of yoga schedule you follow to keep your health and vitality without increasing weight.

General Exercise Schedule

	Warm up	10 to 20 min.
A.	Standing position	10 to 20 min.
(a)	Jogging action	1 min.
(b)	Neck rotation	5 round clock and anti clock wise
(c)	Arm circling	-Do-
(d)	Arm swinging	10 rounds clock and anti clock - wise
(e)	Side bending	10 counts each side
(f)	Back front bending	10 counts
(g)	Touching of opposite feet	10 times

(B) Sitting Position:

(a) Feet stretching from ankle joint	10 count each side
(b) Ankle rotation	-do-
(c) Half butterfly	-do-
(d) Full butterfly	-do-
(e) Hand clenching	-do-
(f) Wrist rotation	-do-
(g) Knee rotation	-do-
(h) Chakki chalana	-do-
(C) Lying position	10 count each side
(a) Cycling action of legs	10 count each side
(b) Leg rotation	10 count each side
(c) 30°, 60°, 90° hold of each leg	10 count each side
(d) Side stretching	20 sec. each side

Surya Namaskar

Stay according to capacity

Standing

- *Tad asana*
- *Vriksh asana*
- *Trikon asana* with variations
- *Kati chakra asana*

Sitting:

- Happy posture (sukhasana)
- Lotus Posture (padam asana)
- Parvat asana (smountain pose)
- Half lotus pose
- Cow posture (gomukh asana)
- Vajra asana
- Sujet Vajra asana
- Vakra asana
- Ardhmatsy asana
- Matsya asana
- Aakran dhanur asana

Lying:

- Prone position
- Bhujang asana
- Dhanur asana
- Ardh ghalbhasana

- Shalbh asana

Spine

- Sarvang asana
- Vipreet kami
- Hal asana
- Chakra asana

Facial exercises:

Movement of eye balls to different directions such as

Up down

- Round clockwise and anti clockwise
- Make cross with eye balls
- Gazing at near and far objects
- Blinking etc.

Raising eyebrows

- Engulf the air in mouth and breathe it
- Art
- Pressing the jaws
- Rubbing the ears
- Face massage etc.

Pranayamas - 5 min. to 30 min.

- Correct breathing – sitting and lying
- Anulom –vilom pranayama
- Nadishodhan pranayama
- Ujjayi pranayama
- Shitati/sheetkari pranayama
- Yoga nidra

It should, however, be realized that yoga will not give overnight results nor will its benefits be achieved easily. Only regular practices will bring relief. The importance of yoga is that it provides relief from many diseases and symptoms without using any medicine. It also helps in preventing many diseases and consequently obviates the potential use of medicines for treating those diseases. Thus yoga is an important part of demedicalization. Moreover, the practice of yoga is an integral part of Indian culture. It gets intimately integrated with our way of life and daily routine. Above all, it does not require any dependence on others except for initial training by a yoga guru. After that the individual has to practice and continue with it.

41

Self Care by Women Having Bronchial Asthma

Sukhpal Kaur, D Behera, D Gupta and SK Verma

Asthma affects people of all ages and being a chronic disease is an important health problem. Despite the improvement in understanding about various aspects of asthma, its incidence, morbidity and mortality has increased worldwide.[1,2] Several factors that can explain this phenomenon include genetic predisposition; exposure to cockroach allergens, house dust mites and tobacco smoke. Lack of asthma education and nonexistence or lack of access to asthma support groups prevents the asthma patients and their families from getting easy relief from the avoidable suffering. High levels of non-compliance to recommended treatment in asthma patients is another important practical problem.[3-5]

Most of the allergens responsible for asthma are probably prevalent inside the house since this is the place where human beings spend most of their lives. Exposures to allergens originating from pet animal at home is one of the most readily preventable immediate hazard at home.[6] Drug allergy is present in a good number of asthmatics and many commonly used drugs are also known to cause severe and even fatal exacerbations of asthma.[7] For those patients on inhalators, many studies have shown poor inhalation techniques.[8-15] These various problems in bronchial asthma can be minimized if not eliminated, if bronchial asthma patients are made aware of the disease in general with special emphasis on their treatment related individual requirements. Patient empowerment can go a long way in better patient management if they are taught self-management of asthma.

Bailey et al.[16] and Wilson et al.[17] examined the effects of asthma education programs. In the Bailey study, the treatment group showed increased adherence and functional status. The education group in the Wilson study showed improvement in metered dose inhaler technique, environmental control measures and reported symptoms.

The ultimate goals and objectives of asthma self-management programs are:

- Fewer days' absence from school or work
- Improved school or work performance
- Fewer trips to the emergency room (ER)
- Fewer unscheduled doctors' office visits or hospital stays.
- Improved level of general health.
- Fewer, shorter, and less severe asthmatic episodes.

These goals and objectives could be achieved by conveying to the asthma patients information about the disease itself; by training and giving some practice in skills like trigger identification and avoidance, diaphragmatic breathing, postural drainage, and relaxation and stress reduction. Doctors and nurses only have the opportunity to influence patient decision during clinical contact, i.e., every 30 or perhaps 90 days. It is unlikely that a piece of advice given in a consultation will be followed every day for the following 30 or 90 days. Therefore, written information accessible to patients on a daily basis is essential. The major problem in asthma care is translating the theory of good asthma care into every day practice: self-management plans represent the best available option to do this.[18,19]

A study was conducted by the authors in which a **Self Care Manual on Bronchial Asthma** was prepared. A total of 523 diagnosed bronchial asthma patients were enrolled. Out of these

260 patients were included in the study group to whom self-care manual was given and 263 were included in the control group to whom no specific instructions were given. After the initial interview (0 week), follow up of all the patients was carried out at the intervals of two weeks, six months and one year. Various parameters studied were - knowledge of the patients regarding the disease, their symptomatology, emotional reactions, various triggering factors which were inducing and / or precipitating symptoms, the self-care measures they adopted at the time of severe attacks and the indices of asthma morbidity during the last one year. Around 60% of the patients were females. A significantly higher number of study group patients showed a significant improvement in knowledge, symptom and emotion scores at all the three post-intervention visits. There was no relationship of disease severity with the knowledge of the subjects in both the groups. However, there was a statistically significant relationship of disease severity with the symptoms and emotions in both the groups i.e. the symptoms and emotions increased with the severity of the disease. Irrespective of the disease severity the knowledge scores were higher; while the symptoms and the emotion scores were lower after intervention. The number of subjects whose symptoms were induced and/or precipitated by exposure to various triggering factors was significantly reduced in study group subjects for all the triggers. However, in the control group, this trend was there but only for a few triggers.

There was no significant difference between study and control groups (both before and after intervention) in the attitude regarding the self-care and the medical help they sought during an acute attack of asthma although the number of subjects who had acute attack(s) at last follow up (1 year) were very few as compared to the number at the beginning of the study in both the groups. Significantly more subjects in study group acquired the desirable position of sitting with forward leaning during an acute attack. Also, significantly, more subjects from study group at 1 year practiced breathing exercises during an acute attack as compared to control subjects. There was a statistically significant decrease in the number of severe attacks, number of emergency visits and need of injections during last 1 year in both the groups, though the differences were more marked in study group. However, there was a significant decrease in hospital admissions and absence from school /or job only in study group at 1 year as compared to control group. All the subjects read the booklet (self-care manual) at least once or more. All of them could understand it; found the language easy and found it to be useful for them. (The manual text is enclosed).

Self care manual on bronchial asthma What is asthma?

Asthma is a chronic inflammatory disorder of the airways in which the bronchi or air passages are swollen or narrowed. As the air passages become smaller, free flow of air is hampered. It affects people of all ages, can be severe, and sometimes can be fatal. We call this problem as '*dama*' in local language...simply put, it is breathlessness problem.

How asthma develops?

In the patients with bronchial asthma, the airways are hyper-responsive to certain stimuli. Exposure to these stimuli brings about an attack of asthma in the following ways:

1. The muscles in the walls of airways undergo constrictions. (Fig. 1.1)
2. There is swelling of airways. (Fig. 1.2)

These various events reduce the airway caliber and the airflow through them.

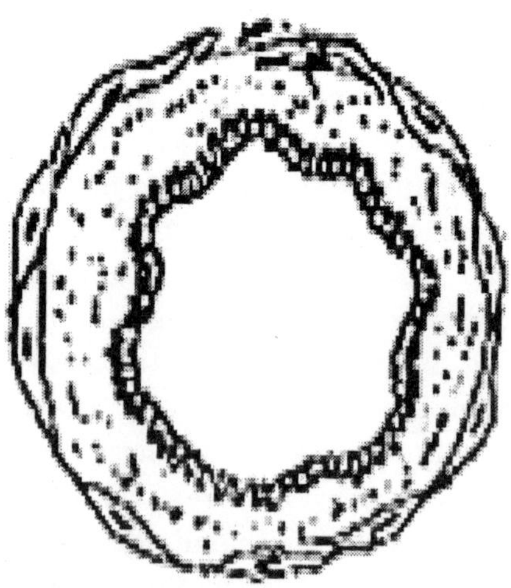

Fig 1.1Breathing tube in a normal person.

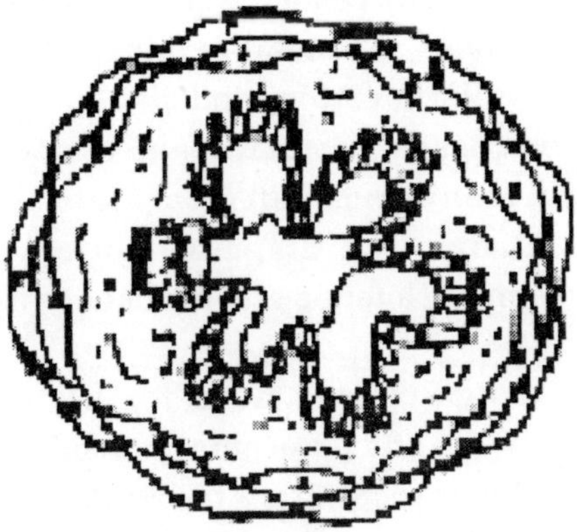

FiG. 1.2. Breathing tube during asthma.

What are the triggering factors in bronchial asthma?

The triggering factors or the stimuli, which brings about an attack of asthma, vary from person to person and time to time. A few common factors could be:-

1. **Allergens:** Allergen is a substance, which brings about hypersensitivity or a reaction in the susceptible persons. For other persons, these allergens may be harmless. The various allergens causing bronchial asthma are as follows: (Fig. 2.1 to Fig. 2.8)
   - (a) **House dust:** The major allergen in the house dust is the fecal matter of dust mite. High concentration is found in dust on mattresses, pillows, curtains, carpets, books, papers, and soft toys etc. Other allergens in house are animal dander and feathers.
   - (b) **Pollens**: Plant pollen grains cause seasonal attacks of asthma during pollination season (September to October and March to April)
   - (c) **Domestic pets:** Dogs, cats etc.
   - (d) **Insects**: like cockroaches etc.
   - (e) **Fungi and molds:** Fungus on walls and other organic matter release its spores in the air, which could be responsible for asthma.
   - (f) **Tobacco smoke:** Both active as well as passive smoke.
   - (g) **Various dusts:** While sifting/cleaning pulses and cereals etc.

(h) **Air pollutants:** Smoke from wood, factories, crackers, incense sticks, vehicular exhaust

(i) **Fabrics:** Wool, cotton, and silk etc.

(j) **Odours:** Soaps, perfumes, and cosmetic etc.

(k) **Drugs**: Many drugs can precipitate asthma attacks —

- Some drugs like disprin, brufen, indomethacin, piroxicam, diclofenac etc. commonly used for pain and fever.
- Some drugs mainly used for high blood pressure (propranolol) and glaucoma (timolol) etc.

3. **Infections:** Upper respiratory tract infections (usually viral infections) like common cold, sinus (air filled cavities around nose) infection and sore throat, can also precipitate an attack of asthma.

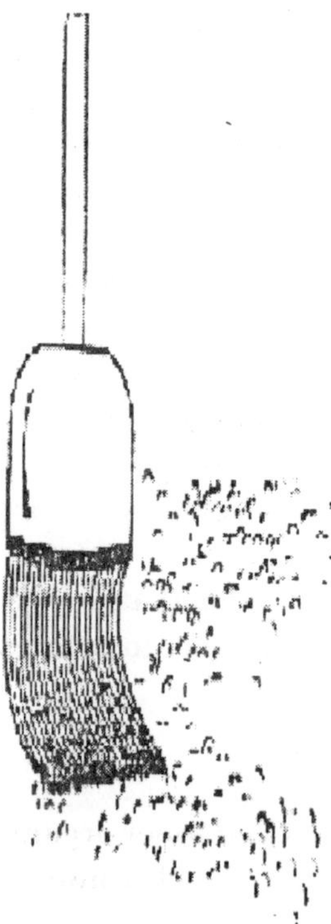

Dust while sweeping
Fig. 2.1

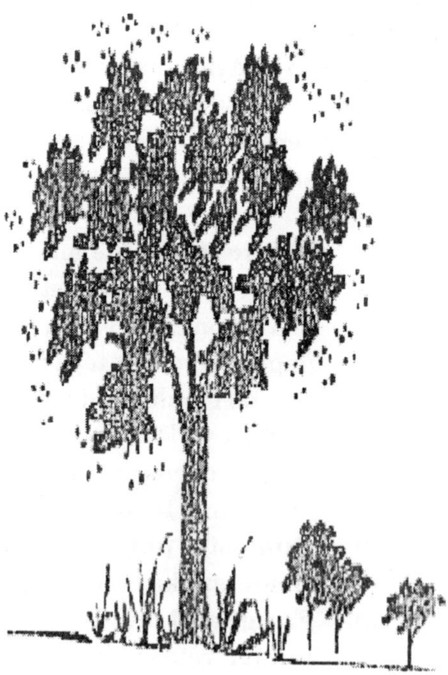

Pollens
Fig. 2.2

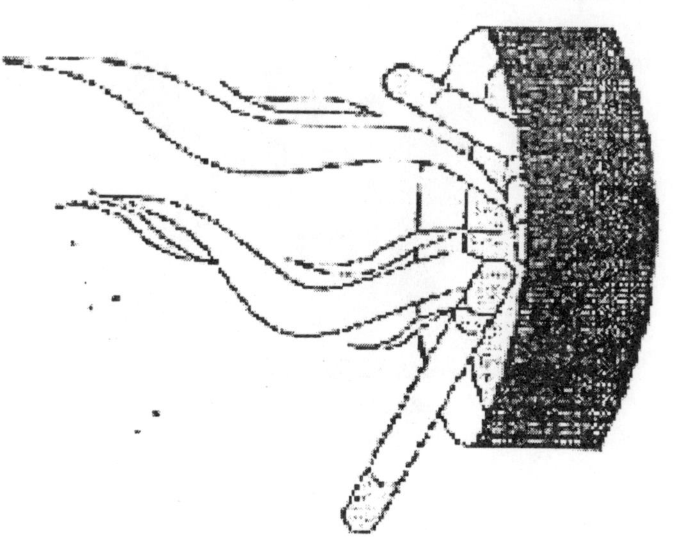

Cigarette smoking
Fig. 2.3

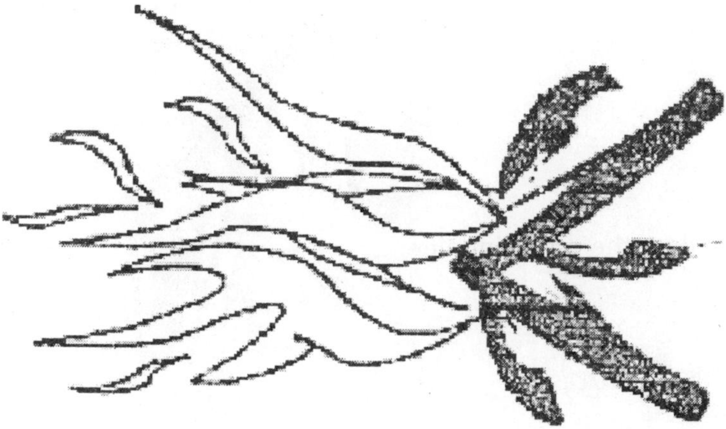

Wood smoke
Fig. 2.4

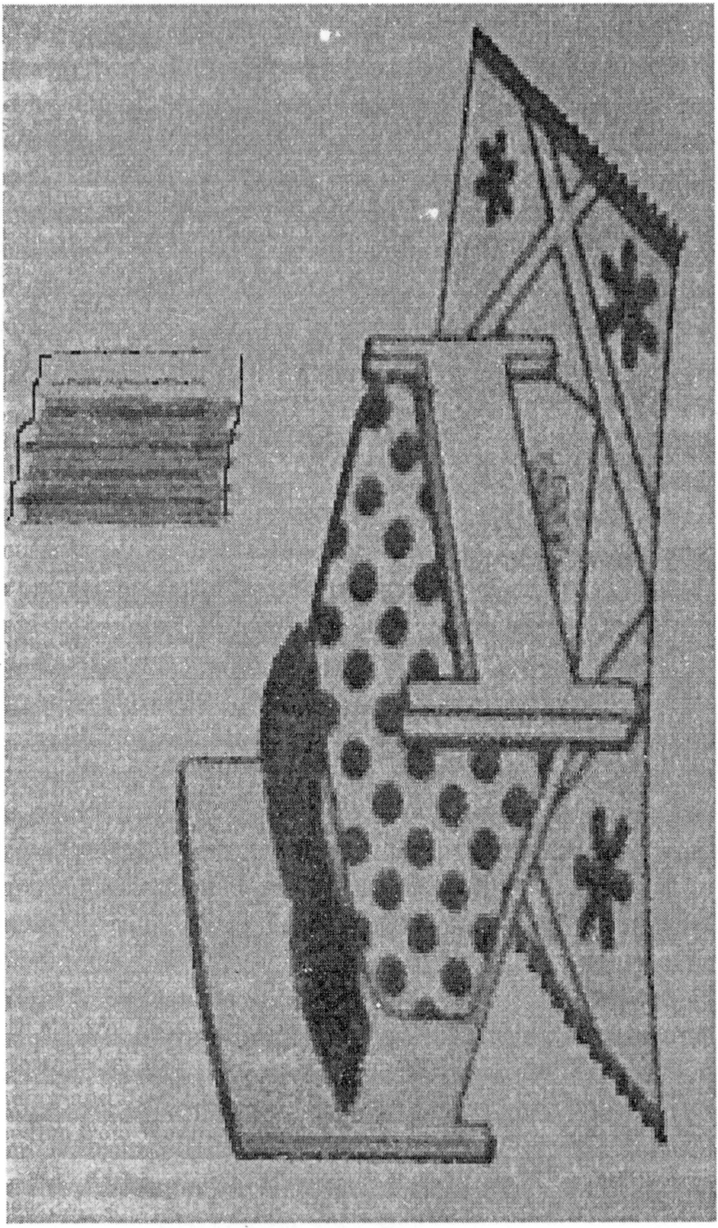

Dust of pillows, curtains, carpets and mattresses
(Fig. 2.5)

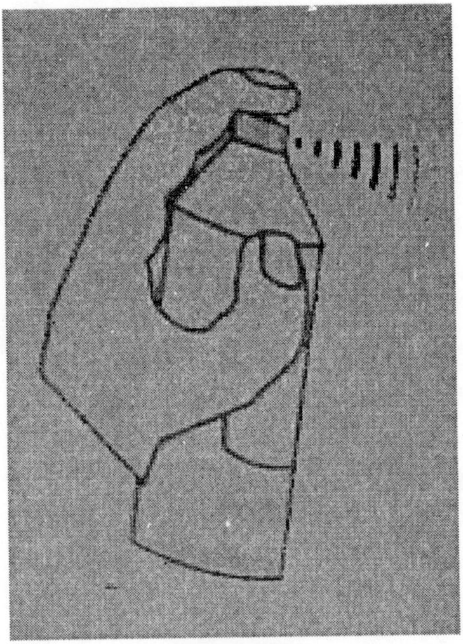

Perfumes
(Fig. 2.6)

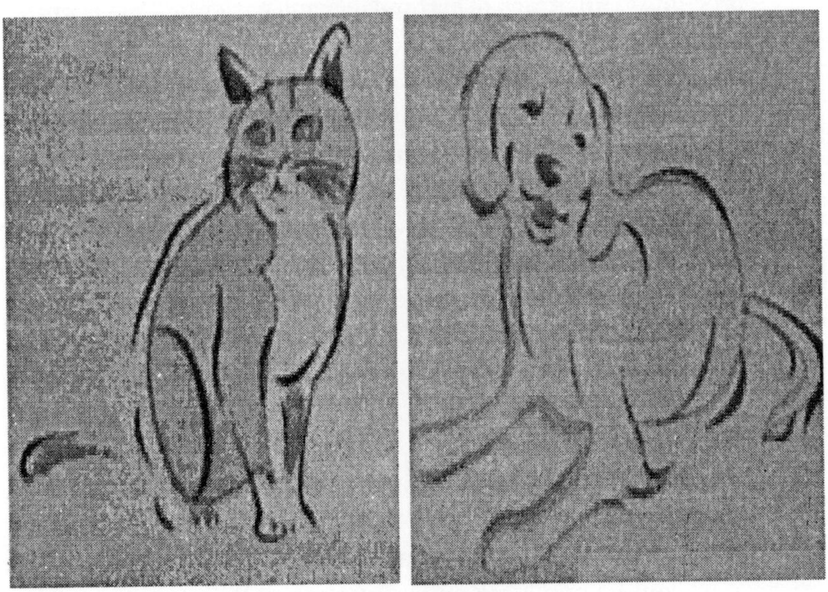

Animal with fur
(Fig. 2.7)

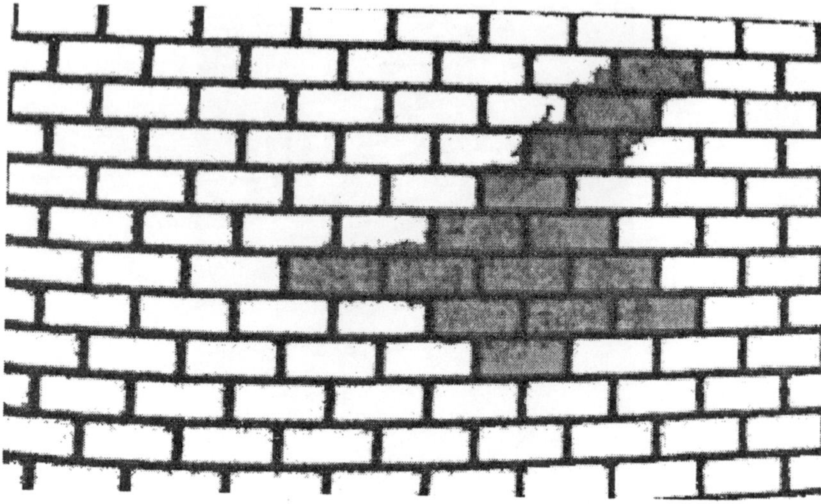

Fungus on wall (Fig. 2.8)

3. **Emotions:** Sometimes laughter, excitement, anger and mental tension may trigger an attack of asthma.
4. **Exercise:** Heavy physical activity, excessive exercise can precipitate an attack of asthma in some patients. This is known as exercise induced asthma (EIA).
5. **Occupational asthma:** In this form, symptoms appear towards the end of the working day and improve at the weekend or holidays. A partial list of hazardous professions includes carpenters, millers, painters, farmers, flour mill workers, detergent factory workers etc.
6. **Certain disease conditions:** Like reflux of acid from stomach into food pipe are known to precipitate asthma.

What are the signs and symptoms of asthma?

1. Shortness of breath
2. Tightness in chest
3. Wheezing (musical sounds during respiration)
4. Cough

These symptoms could be seasonal, after physical activity like exercise or could come after exposure to the allergens.

At a given time all the symptoms may or may not be present in a particular patient.

Management of asthma

Is asthma curable?

There is no permanent cure for asthma, but the suffering can be substantially minimized if one takes care of the following things:

- Avoid allergens and known triggers.
- Take medicines as per doctor's advice.
- Know the warning signs and symptoms of the disease.

What are the general measures that you should observe to manage an attack of asthma?

When you have an attack of asthma —

1. It is desirable to sit in an upright position with an adequate support.
2. You should not try to force out the air from your lungs.
3. It is useful to maintain a calm attitude and there should be no environmental disturbances.
4. Adequate fluid intake helps in expectoration of sputum and prevents dehydration.
5. You should not use sedatives during an attack of asthma.
6. Try to identify different triggering factors, so that, if possible you can avoid these in future.

How to face tension, fear and restlessness during an acute attack of asthma?

In some of the patients, worry and restlessness exaggerate the acute attack of asthma. Breathing becomes fast and shallow; severity increases and the inhaled medicine do not reach into lungs. Thus, it is important to control tension and restlessness, so that the inhaled medicine is utilized effectively.

How to control tension?

Concentrating on some specific physical activity like rate of breathing can help to control tension. The increase in respiration due to tension can be decreased by two ways:

1. **Drinking any liquid slowly**: Taking a glass of water or any liquid in hand and drinking slowly can decrease tension in the body by diverting the attention of patient away from

his ailment. Moreover, it is necessary to decrease the respiratory rate to drink any liquid. With the decrease in respiratory rate, bronchodilator (asthalin or tarbutaline) can act more effectively.

2. **Breathing exercises:** Breathing exercises can be performed in the following manner:

- Sit down.
- Take in deep breath while gently pressing your upper abdomen with both of your hands. (Fig. 3.1)
- Take out your breath slowly through the pursed lips (Fig. 3.2)

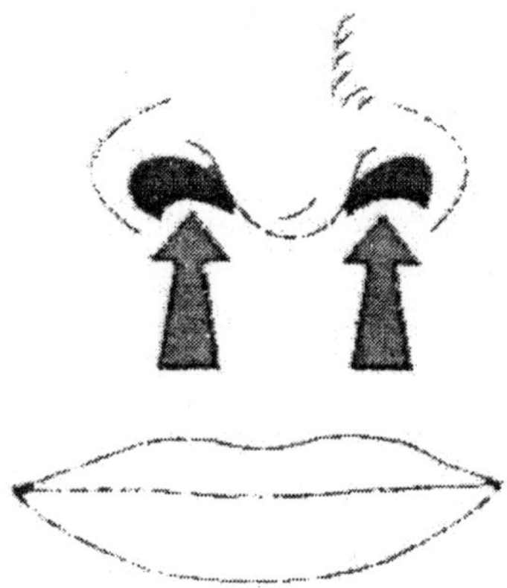

Fig. 3.1

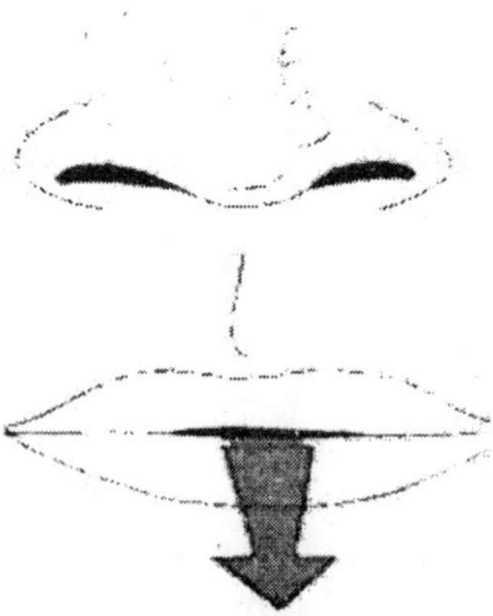

Fig. 3.2

- Repeat the above steps at least twice.
- While performing breathing exercises, use the prescribed inhaler.
- Repeat the steps if needed.

What is an inhaler?

An inhaler is a pump like device filled with asthma medicine under pressure. It delivers very-very small particles of medicine into the lungs. (Fig. 4)

There are some misconceptions regarding the use of inhaler in the general public that:

(a) Inhalers are dangerous to use.

(b) Inhalers are the last resort drugs and nothing else will work later.

(c) Inhalers are habit-forming medicines.

(d) Inhalers damage heart and lungs in the long run.

It needs to be emphasized that these misconceptions are absolutely baseless because

(a) Use of inhaler for the asthmatic patients is not only useful but, in fact, it is the safest way of treatment. Moreover, the side effects seen with oral and injectable drugs do not occur

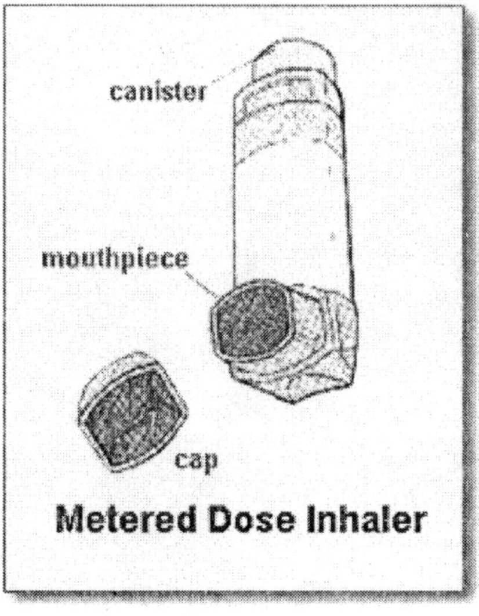

Fig. 4

with inhalers as the dose of the medicine is very low (<1/10th) as compare to oral or injections. Also, the inhaled medicines act directly on the respiratory tract.

(b) Inhalers are, nowadays, the first drugs to be used even in mild asthma.All other medicines used along with inhalers or otherwise fully retain their effects.

(c) Inhalers are not habit forming medicines and do not damage heart and lungs at all.

(d) It must be remembered that inhaled medicines give an immediate relief.

How to use the inhaler correctly?

Inhaler must be used correctly to be effective. The basic steps fro using inhaler are:

1. Remove the cap. (Fig. 4.1). Hold inhaler in an upright position and shake well. (Fig. 4.2)

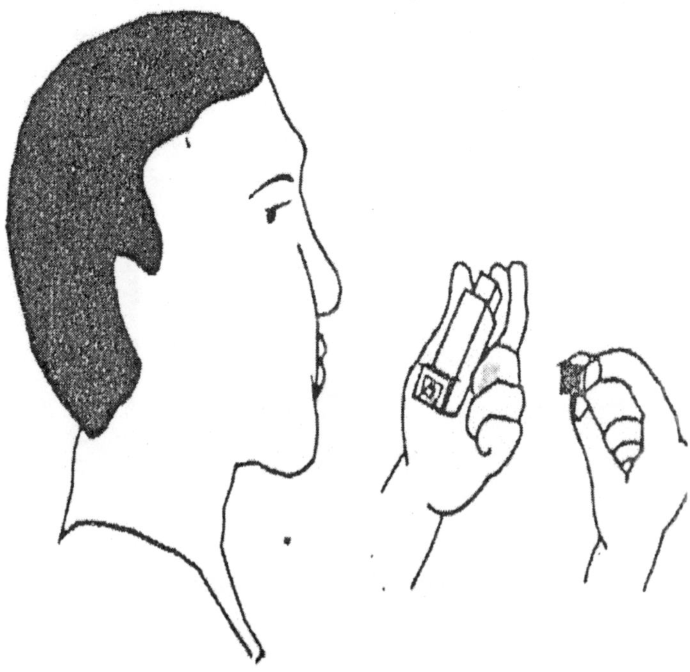

Fig. 4.1

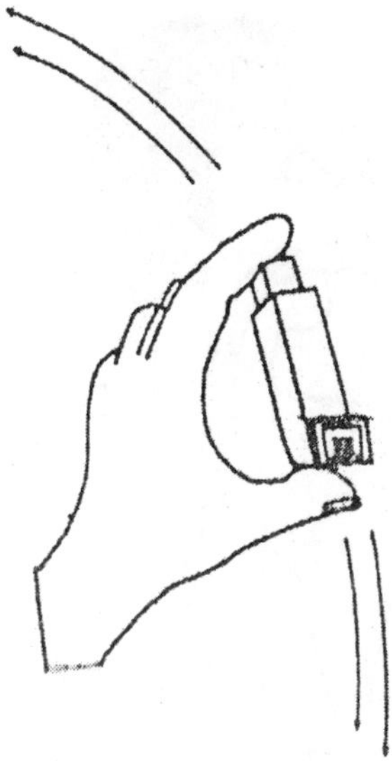

Fig. 4.2

2. Tilt your head back slightly and breathe out slowly. (Fig 4.3)

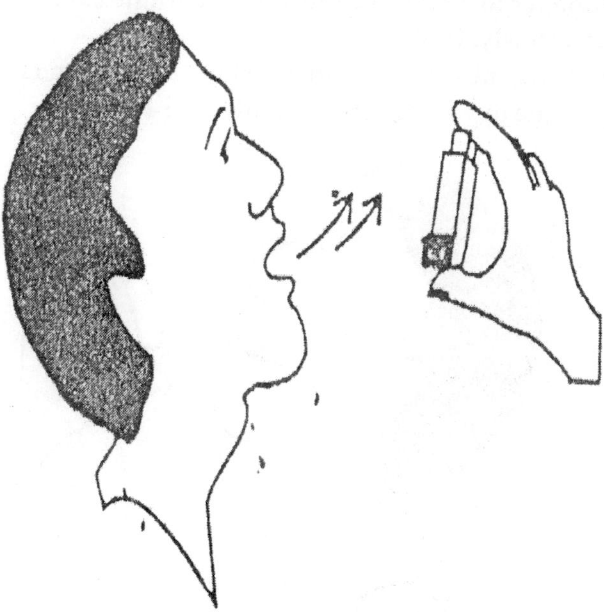

Fig. 4.3

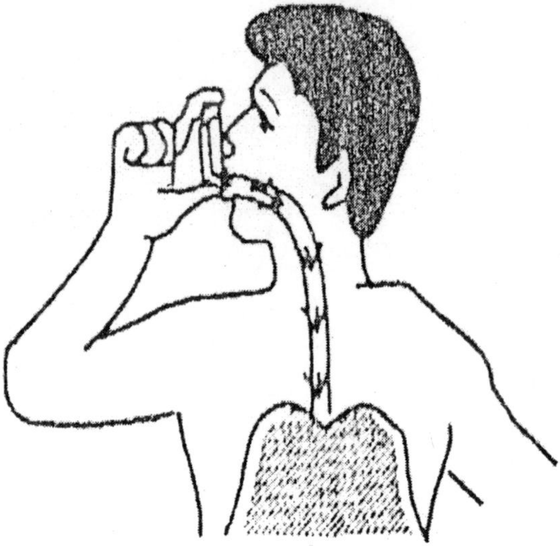

Fig. 4.4

3. Close your lips around mouth piece firmly, start to breathe in slowly through the mouth and simultaneously press the canister to release the doze and continue to breathe in deeply and slowly. (Fig 4.4)
4. Remove inhaler, hold breathe for 5 to 10 seconds (Fig 4.5) and breathe out slowly and steadily (Fig 4.6)

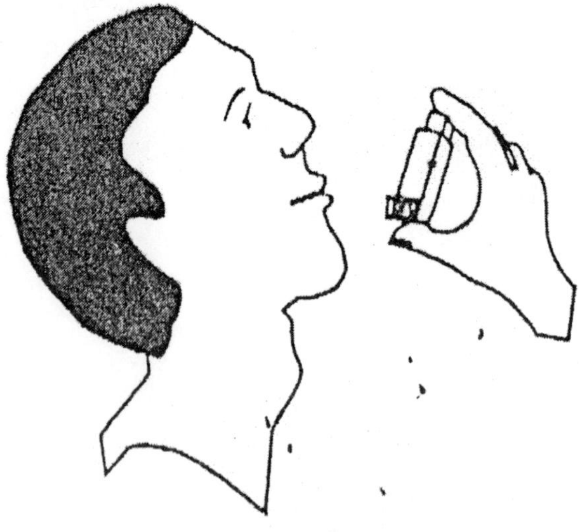

Fig. 4.5

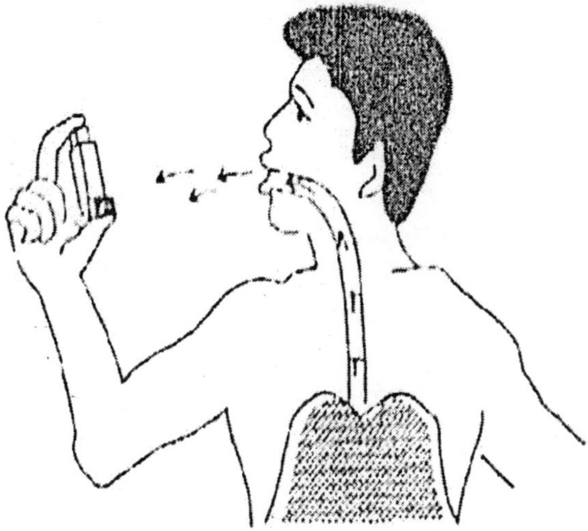

Fig. 4.6

5. If another dose is needed, wait for at least one minute and repeat steps 2 to 4. After use replace the cover on the mouth piece (Fig 4.7)

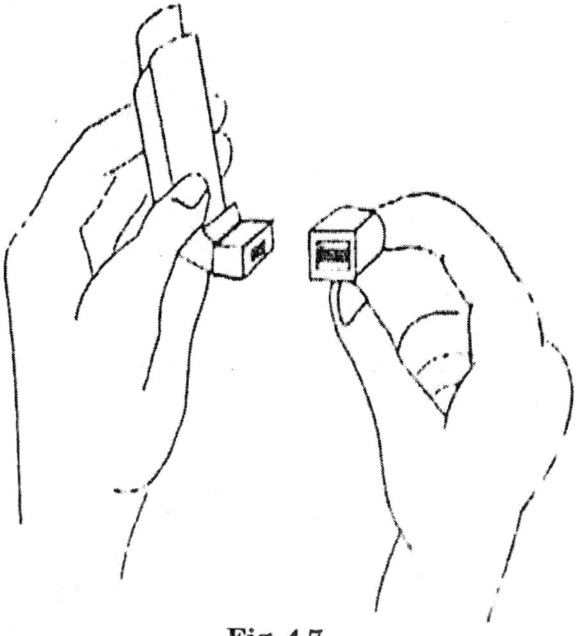

Fig. 4.7

6. Clean the mouth piece regularly (everyday) with warm water.
7. If using a steroid inhaler, rinse your mouth with water after each use to prevent excess deposition of drug in your oral cavity.

Important points to remember:

1. Do not rush steps 2 and 3. It is important that you begin to breathe in slowly through the mouth just before pressing the canister.
2. Keep the protective cover on the mouthpiece while not in use, so that dirt cannot get in.
3. The number of doses is written on the inhaler. However, you must check daily, if medicine is there in the inhaler or not, by pressing the canister.

Preventing Asthma Attacks

1. Keep your house dust free

(a) Bed making, dusting and cleaning of house should be done while the patient is out of room. Regular mopping of the floor should be done with moistened cloth regularly.

(b) If you have to do these tasks, you should wear a face mask.

(c) Keep wall hangings, calendars, and loose papers clean and dust free.

(d) It is better to have minimum of such hangings or loose papers in the house

2. Reducing hazards from house dust mites

(a) Remove carpets from bedroom and avoid unnecessary wall hangings and heavy curtains in the room.

(b) Reduce indoor humidity by letting fresh air and sunlight to come in the room.

(c) Bedclothes and curtains should be washed frequently.(once in 6 months at least)

(d) Keep the books, files and loose papers in the closed almirahs. These should be regularly dusted

(e) Use foam mattresses and pillow instead of cotton ones.

(f) Expose your beddings to sun frequently.

(g) House should be regularly whitewashed/painted (at least once in 3 years)

3. **Preventive measures for pollens**

(a) If the plant responsible for allergy is identified by allergy test or otherwise, then

(i) If possible remove the plant from the surroundings.

(ii) You should shift to another place or city if possible.

(b) Don't move around in the gardens (especially during pollination season).

(c) Use face mask while going out.

(d) If going out by scooter, use face cover and the helmet.

(e) Don't move out of the house before sunrise and after sunset.

(f) Keep the windows and ventilators of your house closed for most of the time.

(g) Mop your house twice daily-morning and evening, using a moistened cloth.

(h) Avoid going out during the harvesting season.

4. **Preventive measures for molds:** February to April and then July to December i.e. the rainy periods and months thereafter are the important periods for taking precautions against molds. Following measures can help avoiding exposures to molds:

(a) There should be no dampness in the rooms.

(b) Rooms should get adequate sunlight and ventilation.

(c) Use mask while cleaning the walls.

(d) Old furniture and other waste articles should not be kept for long at any place in the house.

(e) Keep your desert cooler clean and change the pads before use every year.

(f) Avoid entering the room which has been lying closed for a long period.

5. **Prevention from animal allergens and animal dander**

(a) Remove pet animals from the house. If they cannot be removed from the house, keep them away from your room.

(b) Bathe your pet frequently which may reduce the amount of dander.

(c) Avoid caressing pet animals.

6. **Prevention from indoor irritants:**

(a) Avoid exposure to wood smoke and tobacco smoke.

(b) Avoid exposure to strong odors and sprays such as perfume, powder, room deodorizers, fresh paint etc.

7. Prevention from some other allergens

Patients should not come in contact with the dust arising from cleaning of wheat, pulses, wool and cotton, if their symptoms are triggered by these allergens. Similarly, one can avoid the symptoms caused because of the smoke due to wood, factories, crackers and incense sticks. Asthma caused due to the strong odor of soap, perfume, and powder etc. can also be avoided in the same manner.

If egg, fish and milk etc. are observed as a cause of asthma these items should not be consumed.

8. Prevention of respiratory tract infection

(a) Avoid contact with a person, who has infection of respiratory tract.

(b) In case of respiratory tract infection consult your doctor for further treatment.

9. Prevention of occupational asthma

If the symptoms are induced by exposure to the dust at place of work, one should work in the dust free environment, if possible. But, if due to some reasons it is necessary to work at that place, one should use mask or any other cloth to cover the nose and mouth.

Is asthma familial ?

In certain people, there may be predisposition to allergic disorders (atopy) like frequent cold, eczema etc. Children of the asthmatic patients have more chances of developing asthma in the life. Chances of a child to become an asthmatic are 25-50% if one parent is asthmatic and around 50-75% if both the parents are asthmatics. Except for taking the preventive measures against the triggering factors, probably nothing much can be done to change such predisposition of a patient.

Smoking and asthma

Tobacco smoke is a powerful irritant and has a harmful effect. Smoke from the people's cigarettes (passive smoking) should also be avoided.

Exercise and asthma

If the symptoms are induced due to certain exercises or heavy exertion, one should always use preventive medicines a few minutes before exposure to these.

Remember

1. Asthma is not caused by psychological factors only.
2. People with asthma can live full and active life.
3. Asthma is not an infectious disease.
4. If proper treatment is taken, you will remain symptom free and you are like any other normal person.
5. Always carry your quick-relief medicine with you when you leave home. And it will help if you also carry a card in your pocket with your address, phone no. and instructions to use of inhaler if a situation arises that you need any help of the bystanders .

References

1. Robertson CF, Heycock E, Bishop J, Nolan P, Olinsky A. and Phelan PD. Prevalence of asthma in Melbourne school children: changes over 26 years. B.M.J. 1991; 302:116-118.
2. Ninan TK and Russell G. Respiratory symptoms and atopy in Aberdeen school children: evidence from two surveys 25 years apart. B.M.J. 1992; 304: 873-875.
3. Taggert VS, Zuckerman AE and Lucas S et al. Adapting a self-management education program for asthma for use in out patient clinic. Ann. Allergy 1987; 58: 173-178.
4. Taggert VS, Zuckerman AE and Sly RM et al. You can control asthma: evaluation of an asthma education program for hospitalized inner-city children. Patient Educa. Council 1991; 17: 5-47.
5. Watts RW, McLennai G, Bassham I and el-Saadi O. Do patients with asthma fill their prescriptions? A primary compliance study. Australian Family Physician 1997; 26: 4-6.
6. Sporik R, Holgate SD, Platus–Mills TAE et al. Exposure to housedust mite allergens (Der P1) and development of asthma in childhood. N. Eng. J. Med 1990; 323: 502-507.

7. Gupta SK. Clinical profile of bronchial asthma in Eastern India-A prospective analysis of 7208 patients. Lung India 1996; 14: 60-65.
8. Epstein SW, Manning CD, Ashley MJ. and Corey PN. Survey of the clinical use of pressurized aerosol inhalers. Can. Med. Assoc. J. 1979; 120: 813-816.
9. Lindgren S, Bake B and Larsson S. Clinical consequences of inadequate inhalation technique in asthma therapy. Eur. J. Respir. Dis. 1987; 70:93-98.
10. Pedersen S, Frost L and Arnfred T. Errors in inhalation technique and efficiency in inhaler use in asthmatic children. Allergy 1986; 41: 118-124.
11. Ellul-Micallef R, Moren F, Wetterlin K and Hidinger KG. Use of a special inhaler attachment in asthmatic children. Thorax 1980; 35: 620.
12. Lonbardi TP (1987). Cited by Côté J, Kartier A and Robichaud P et al. Influence on asthma morbidity of asthma education programs based on self-management plans following treatment optimization. Am. J. Respir. Crit. Care Med 1997; 155: 1509-1514.
13. Goldberg IS and Laurenco RV. Deposition of aerosols in pulmonary disease. Arch. Intern. Med 1973; 131: 88.
14. Pedersen, S. Optimal use of tube spacer aerosols in asthmatic children. Ann. Allergy 1985; 15: 473.
15. Dolovich M, Ruffin RE, Roberts R and Newhouse MT. Optimal delivery of aerosols from metered dose inhalers. Chest 1981; 80: 911-915.
16. Bailey W, Richards JJ, Brooks C, Soong S, Windsor R and Manzella B. A randomized trial to improve self-management practices of adults with asthma. Arch. Intern. Med 1990; 150: 1664-1668.
17. Wilson SR, Scamagas P and German DF et al. A controlled trial of two forms of self-management education for adults with asthma. Am. J. Med 1993; 94: 564-576.
18. Brewis RAL. Patient education, self-management plans and peak-flow measurements. Respir. Med 1991; 85: 457-462.
19. Partridge MR. Asthma: Guided self-management. B.M.J. 1994; 308: 547-548.

Index

D

E

I

J

K

L

R

T

U

V